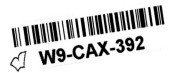
Rewire Your Brain, Rewire Your Life

A HANDBOOK FOR
STROKE SURVIVORS & THEIR CAREGIVERS

Bob Guns, Ph.D.

First Edition 2008
ISBN 978-1-59594-262-3
Library of Congress Control Number:
2008937510

ACKNOWLEDGMENTS

I want to thank all the people who agreed to be interviewed for this handbook. They include eleven stroke survivors and five caregivers. All willingly and openly shared their stories to encourage stroke survivors to stretch themselves a little further to improve the quality of their lives.

I'd also like to acknowledge some of the other key people who helped me launch this project. Inspiration initially came from an article in the periodical, *Neurology Now.* Sharon Begley, science editor of *Newsweek,* reviewed a book entitled **The Brain That Changes Itself** by Dr. Norman Doidge.

That review and my subsequent reading of the book opened a new world of hope for me and, I believed, for other stroke survivors. Begley and Doidge both stated that neuroscience showed the brain as *neuroplastic.* It was far more malleable and changeable than we thought. It was not hard-wired after all.

What a breakthrough! And what hope that represented for those of us who had suffered a stroke or brain injury. If we stimulated the brain properly, maybe we could do a little more to regain some of our lost capability. I want to thank both of these science 'investigators' for indirectly inspiring me to write this handbook.

I'd like to thank two neurologists and one brain surgeon for ensuring 'the brain' parts of the handbook were on the mark: Dr. Larry Goldstein, Dr. Andrew Braunstein, and Dr. Jeffrey Yablon.

My wife and caregiver, Veronica, kept challenging me in clarifying and configuring what I was trying to write. What a gal! Our daughter, Laura McLafferty, made her own wonderful contribution by suggesting a creative idea for the cover, then photographing it. She is a budding photographer, and the front cover clearly demonstrates her talent.

My stroke support group in Mooresville, NC kindly put up with my latest rantings about the brain and neuroplasticity. What a support group!

I have to give a special thanks to the engaging 80 year-old Charles Memrick (with his 'team' of caregivers) for volunteering to be the first RAISE 'self-improver.' One of Charles' first comments: "Well, what credentials do you have to put me through this?" Good question. I hope I answered it.

TABLE OF CONTENTS

Why the handbook was written; the case for hope for stroke survivors; and overview of the handbook's content and format.

A profile of Strong Stroke Survivors and eleven personal stories (from interviews) that illustrate five major characteristics of Strong Stroke Survivors:

Caregivers can make the difference in a stroke survivor's survival and quality of life (and I can vouch for that). They can also play a key role in the three week self-improvement program (RAISE) the survivor is about to undertake. Five perspectives on the caregiver's role (again, based on interviews) are presented.

Fourth Section: Rebuilding Capability

Outlines the planning and action-taking part of the handbook. The five step process helps the survivor and caregiver select an appropriate capability to work on, put together a plan to raise that capability, and act on it:

1. **R**eflect
2. **A**nalyze
3. **I**dentify
4. **S**tart
5. **E**valuate

Provides two real world examples of RAISE programs that worked—the author's and a Strong Stroke Survivor's, both with exceptional outcomes. A Bibliography, Stroke Associations, Stroke Support Websites, and Alternative Therapies are also included.

First Section
WHY THERE IS HOPE

"Pick yourself up, dust yourself off.
Start all over again."
(music by Jerome Kern, lyrics by Dorothy Fields)

Guiding Question:

What is the basis for hope?

Rewire Your Brain, Rewire Your Life is written for *stroke survivors who haven't seen improvement in capability for some time, and likely haven't been working at it.* So the idea of the handbook is to get you 'off the bench and back in the game.' Along with your caregiver.

- ***You willing to try?***

This document is first of all a handbook. You will be asked to participate- AND PRACTICE. Hands on. We're after some improvement here. If you're willing to try once again, this is the handbook for you. Step forward and make something happen. Get your hands dirty and worry about washin' em' later.

- ***Does this describe you? If not, you're reading the wrong handbook.***

Recent research (especially by Taub and Merzenich) suggests that most who have suffered a traumatic brain injury or stroke **can** enhance their capability even some time after their stroke. Taub, for example, had one patient, who 50 years after his stroke, undertook therapy that significantly improved his capability.

Another researcher, Bach-y-Rita, suggested that about six months after a stroke, the brain likely needs time to rewire and consolidate all the rapid, radical restructuring and learning it has gone through. The brain has to pause before it undertakes its next round of learning and rewiring.

Bach-y-Rita's point is that this period of consolidation doesn't mean more improvement can't take place- it just might take longer. Believing that improvement ends at this point is a misconception. Unfortunately, too many stroke survivors do believe they're tapped out. According to recent research and therapy techniques, not necessarily so.

- *Are you tapped out? Or do you believe you can still improve?*

Ratey and others contend that ... "There are many documented cases in which patients who have sustained brain or spinal-cord damage have shown significant improvement." (Ratey, *A User's Guide to the Brain,* p. 167) Moreover, "The brain's ability to rewire means in principle that it can recover from damage." (Ratey, p. 38)

This handbook, therefore, is targeted at longer term stroke survivors. In the final sections, you will design a three week plan to improve your capability—not just on your own, but in tandem with your caregiver(s).

- *"I have to put together a plan? Oh, oh, that's a lot of work." Well, are you prepared to do that work?*

All suggestions in this handbook have actually been tried and successfully implemented by the author (who is himself a stroke survivor) and his caregiver. Moreover, a growing number of people have already implemented their RAISE plans and achieved significant results.

Although this handbook is based on the notion that most stroke survivors can continue to increase their capability, many therapists and doctors tend to 'give up' about six months after a stroke. Therapy health insurance usually has run out. Moreover, many stroke survivors themselves don't think they're capable of improving beyond their initial recovery.

This handbook disagrees with that notion. Most stroke survivors, with a positive attitude, motivation, and clear focus can indeed improve. Simply put, they need to apply some of the new therapy ideas and techniques based on the brain's flexibility or neuroplasticity.

> Researchers are exploring the brain's own natural capacities to repair nerve damage. Neuroplasticity is a new term that describes the ability of nerve cells to change and modify their activity in responses to changes in the environment.
>
> (Ratey, p. 167)

So, the workbook is laid out in four sections and an Appendix:

- First Section: **Why There Is Hope**
- Second Section: **Strong Stroke Survivors**
- Third Section: **Powerful Caregivers**
- Fourth Section: **Rebuilding Your Capability**
- Appendix: **Examples, Bibliography, Resources for Survivors and Caregivers**

Here's a more specific outline of the workbook and 'map' for your journey to enhanced capability:

First Section: Why There Is Hope

Hope encourages survivors to try things they may not have tried otherwise. All they need is a reason for hope. Sometimes science can provide that reason.

Development of new brain-imaging devices began to show how malleable and flexible the brain actually was, that the brain has the potential to re-learn things lost to stroke. That's the reason for hope and the reason for this handbook.

Second Section: Strong Stroke Survivors

The **Second Section** introduces the idea of strong stroke survivors and their characteristics- supported by some of their stories. In this section you should reflect on your own characteristics and behaviors as a stroke survivor, how they compare with other strong stroke survivors, and how you can build upon them.

What are common characteristics and behaviors these folks hold in common? Here are the ones the author has identified:

- **Realistic**
- **Optimistic and Motivated**
- **Purposeful and Determined**
- **Focused and Disciplined**
- **Resilient**

Third Section: Powerful Caregivers

The **Third Section: Powerful Caregivers** complements the **Second Section: Strong Stroke Survivors**. Each builds on the other's strengths. They need one another.

It's hard to overestimate the importance of caregivers to stroke survivors. Their role is fundamental in co-generating any survivor's plan for enhanced capability.

Five Powerful Caregivers present their views on how to support and coach a stroke survivor.

One stroke survivor told me recently he would only work on improving his capability if somebody else clearly showed he or she cared. So caregivers should be reading this handbook along with stroke survivors. In that way they prepare themselves to be better coaches to their survivors.

Fourth Section: Rebuilding Capability

The handbook's **Fourth Section** is based on the idea of **RAISE**- verb transitive, 'set upright, cause to stand up, **rouse, restore to life'** (The Concise Oxford Dictionary). That's what we're trying to do here- **rouse and restore!**

RAISE will outline the following steps of your self-improvement. I'll be asking you to **reflect** on what happened; **analyze** your present capability; **identify** what you want to work on; **start** to work on it; and finally **evaluate** how you did, and what the next steps are. Each section will focus on one of the **RAISE** steps:

1. **R**eflect
2. **A**nalyze
3. **I**dentify
4. **S**tart
5. **E**valuate

You will complete each of these steps so you can put together a three week plan to improve one specific capability. If you *do* each step in sequence you will be more able to successfully complete your plan to rebuild capability. Is that worth it? You betcha. **RAISE yourself up!**

Appendices

Appendix A: Examples of Action Plans

These personal action plans provide examples drawn from the author's own experience and that of a strong stroke survivor's in constructing and implementing such a plan. These examples will help stroke survivors see how to design and carry out their own set of exercises.

Appendix B: Bibliography

Books in the Bibliography range from those on the brain and how it works to brain neuroplasticity, stroke, and neurons and synapses. Most of these books were referenced in the *Analyze* subsection of RAISE.

Appendix C: Stroke Resources

This section outlines a range of resources stroke survivors can draw from that includes a bibliography, associations, websites, and alternative therapies.

OVERALL STRUCTURE

The structure of the handbook is designed for stroke survivors. First of all, it's short in length. Second, concise paragraphs are used. Third, simple language is used.

Learning in small bits. In particular, stroke survivors in the early stages of their recovery will appreciate this feature. Limited energy, endurance and focusing ability make prolonged reading difficult.

Personal Stories

To make the handbook more 'real world,' eleven strong stroke survivor stories will be told. These are not perfect people. But they are each struggling in a difficult world they hadn't chosen. And there are many more of you out there. In fact, you, the reader, may be one of them.

These people were courageous enough to step forward to tell their stories. But they volunteered in order to help other stroke survivors like you.

It's likely at least one of these stories will resonate with your own situation. We know each person's stroke impediments are different from anybody else's. However, let these people, in their own ways, act as models for the rest of us. You will see Strong Stroke Survivor characteristics in each of them.

I ask you to reflect on each story you read and ask yourself:

- What inspires me in this story?
- What have I learned from it that I can apply in my own life?

Guiding Question

Each section and sub-section will start off with a guiding question. The guiding question focuses the reader on the content to be covered. Moreover, it will generate the reader's motivation to find the answer to that question.

Interactive Design

The handbook is designed to be interactive. That is, the reader will be asked a question after reading a few paragraphs. Readers either write their responses down or simply reflect on their responses.

However, writing is encouraged. In that way, the handbook becomes more personal. This process will help the stroke survivor get ready to develop a three week self-improvement plan.

Summary Points

Each section concludes with Summary Points. These Points capture the essence of each section. They remind stroke survivors of what they just read. Summaries address the issue of short-term memory problems so many of us have to deal with.

SUMMARY POINT

- **"Pick (or RAISE) yourself up, dust yourself off. Start all over again."**

Second Section
STRONG STROKE SURVIVORS

"Strength does not come from physical capacity. It comes from indomitable will."
(Mohanda Ghandi)

Guiding Question:

What makes me a Strong Stroke Survivor?

Some stroke survivors increase their capability beyond what they or anybody else expected. Who are these people? What do they hold in common? Based upon interviews I've conducted, stroke survivors I know, and stories I've read in '*Stroke Connection*' they demonstrate certain common characteristics.

- *What common characteristics have you seen in strong stroke survivors?*

Here are characteristics I've identified:

- **Realistic**
- **Optimistic and motivated**
- **Focused and disciplined**
- **Purposeful and determined**
- **Resilient**

These people are still working on their capability. They

have suffered from weaknesses and setbacks that others also experience. However, they stayed with it. They have the right attitude. And for many, it took years to reach their capability as a Strong Stroke Survivor.

Below you will note a set of behaviors that parallel the strong survivor characteristics. These behaviors will give you a more specific idea of what these characteristics mean- and how they're demonstrated in day to day activities.

STRONG STROKE SURVIVORS

Their Characteristics	Their Behaviors
Realistic	Confront and deal with their disabilities and its implications.
Motivated, Optimistic	Expect to increase their capability.
Focused, Disciplined	Practice targeted repetition to improve capability.
Purposeful, Determined	Lead full life with reduced capability.
Resilient	Recover from inevitable setbacks in improving cabability.

The following sub-sections not only provide more information on each of these characteristics, but illustrate them through stories told by Strong Stroke Survivors. You will also get an opportunity to reflect on each one by answering the follow-up questions.

Based upon these characteristics and stories, what could you do to improve your own situation?

Mr. Pete's Story

Part 1

Six strokes and still alive. How could that be? How did he do it? Well, he did do it. And not only is Mr. Pete still alive but... but I'm getting ahead of myself.

One day in 1993 Mr. Pete's arm became paralyzed on his left side. He was scared to death. He decided to stay home until his wife arrived to take him to the hospital.

He had suffered a hemorrhagic stroke and had an aneurism at the center of his brain. On the first day, a catheter was inserted. The next day a craniotomy was performed. It was dangerous because all his arteries had to be temporarily blocked off as they clipped the aneurism. However, when he left Columbia Presbyterian he walked home.

Mr. Pete actually felt his first five strokes were "a piece of cake," that he was going to lick this thing. Then in 2001 he had his sixth stroke. That's the one that humbled him.

Mr. Pete and his wife had decided to take a few days off. As he started driving them to Boston, his wife noticed he was weaving across three lanes of traffic. So she drove him back to Columbia Presbyterian in New York.

Although he walked into the hospital, after lying in

bed, he couldn't move, couldn't do anything. Mr. Pete was paralyzed on both sides of his body and could neither speak nor eat.

It took Mr. Pete two or three weeks to recover from the anesthesia alone. Not only were two nurses with him all the time, but his bed kept shifting from horizontal to vertical (it was part of his therapy). He was on morphine and thought he was in a drugstore. Mr. Pete was completely disoriented.

His prognosis was grim. The doctors weren't giving Mr. Pete a lot of hope. 'If you live, you'll be extremely debilitated.' For the first six months Mr. Pete was depressed.

He had a lot of time in bed to reflect and reassess things. He felt he couldn't participate in 'life' the way he wanted to. And he wanted to get better. Mr. Pete asked himself, 'What am I going to do now?' It was as if his very identity had altered. For the next nine months he remained completely paralyzed, then partially paralyzed the following six months. A daunting journey.

In therapy he didn't have a lot of energy and felt he wasn't going to get any better. In a nursing home Mr. Pete practiced pulling himself up from his wheelchair by using a railing on the wall. Eventually he could stand. He told his wife he wanted to go home.

However, while in the nursing home, he encountered Freddy, 'a little Oriental guy.' Freddy was a deliberate and focused therapist who helped turn Mr. Pete's life around. In two weeks Mr. Pete learned how to do a 'transfer' (from bed to chair, from chair to wheelchair, etc.).

Initially in his wheelchair, Mr. Pete was virtually catatonic, but eventually he was able to walk around the block a number of times in a row. The neighbors noticed. People began coming to his door asking Mr. Pete to help a friend or family member who had suffered a stroke.

As Mr. Pete's head began to clear, he looked back on his 'previous' life and realized he hadn't been that happy with what he was doing and where he was going. His wife and two sons- and life itself- were what really mattered. He also felt good when he helped others and wanted to do more of that. His 'life search' had ended. Mr. Pete grew more than he ever had and now feels he's a better person.

(You'll find Part 2 at the end of this section on Strong Stroke Survivors.)

Realistic

*"Because things are the way they are,
things will not stay the way they are."*
(Bertolt Brecht)

Guiding Question:

*What's the key to dealing with
the reality you're facing?*

A stroke survivor has to deal with a lot of reality in a hurry—although not always at the outset. The survivor is likely more confused and befuddled than anything else. When the brain does start to clear, the true nature of the survivor's condition begins to sink in.

And what a reality! Radically changed medical condition, work and financial situation, and even relationships—all at once. Such trauma would be difficult for anybody who is close to 'normal,' but somebody whose brain has just been attacked battles uphill on all these issues.

Fortunately, dealing with all this 'stuff' is usually a shared responsibility. A caregiver is likely close at hand to make most of the initial decisions. However, the stroke survivor needs to be brought into the decision-making as soon as possible. Strong survivors accept the 'reality' of their situation more quickly than others. They also want to take back control as soon as possible and take action on some of the more pressing issues.

However, even the strongest have their weak moments and difficulties facing some of the 'reality' that's been flung at them.

- ***What was the most difficult issue you had to face in the early going?***
- ***How did you handle it?***

Janice's Story

A lawyer who could no longer practice as a lawyer. That's painful. A stroke and seizure got in the way.

Janice Rodriguez now works as a volunteer at a speech therapy center. Her family is more important than it ever was. She has balance in her life, but it took a while to get there. Hours and hours of speech therapy and practice to deal with her aphasia and apraxia.

About six o'clock at night, she had been discussing a brief with a partner in her law firm. Suddenly she started feeling weird. Janice had no idea what was going on. She had to go back to her office, but felt as if she were really, really drunk. At first she thought she had been poisoned, so threw away her can of soda.

Finally, when she talked with her husband on the phone, he knew something was wrong and called the main number of her office for help. Then in the emergency room she had a brain seizure. After a CT scan, she was diagnosed as having had an ischemic stroke as well as the seizure. The diagnosis of aphasia and apraxia came later.

She ended up at the National Rehabilitation Hospital in DC. A speech therapist told her she would never fully regain her speaking ability. The apraxia was too severe. Janice's response? "That's just ridiculous. That's just wrong." Janice had begun her recovery.

Because writing and talking were critical in her work as a lawyer, Janice needed to regain her speech and ability to write. She saw this as her interim work. She set a goal of returning to work as a lawyer within a year. But it was hard getting there.

Some of her interim work felt like that of a two year old, so she had a long way to go. Fortunately, she had good therapists: one worked on her speech, the other worked on her computer skills.

Although Janice was at home, she practiced her speech skills for about eight hours a day. She also made it a practice to get out in the world again (including shopping). 'Getting out' played a key role in her recovery.

She reached her goal: Janice went back to work as a lawyer. However, she felt something was missing, but wasn't sure what it was. She knew she had to figure it out for herself. Her seizures continued.

Janice maintained her therapy once a week. However,

she began talking with Darlene Robinson about establishing a Stroke Comeback Center focused on speech therapy for stroke survivors. She left her work as a lawyer. The Center opened in 2005 and now serves about fifty patients a week. Janice works as a volunteer administrator there.

Janice had had to deal with grief about losing all those things she used to do. And she had to allow that grief to happen. Then she decided to come back and fight a different battle. Not only does Janice work at the Center, but she also started a stroke support group.

Janice had finally reached her point of acceptance: "I'm not perfect. But I'm pretty okay."

- *In what ways are you similar to Janice? How are you different?*

- *If you admire what Janice achieved, what would you need to do to be more like Janice?*

Realistic stroke survivors confront and deal with their disability and its implications. They'll gather as much information as they can about their disability, prospects for improvement, and next steps. It also means realistic stroke survivors (eventually) accept their reduced competence but will not accept their inability to do something about it.

- *How realistic are you? What particular things do you accept?*

- *What particular things do you want to work on?*

Mary Lou's Story

Mary Lou's key to recovery? Facing reality. Here's her story.

In 2002, Mary Lou Puls, now 64, had just gotten into her car to go see her son. She went into a roadside restroom and fell on the floor. After her week-long initial recovery in a hospital, she was transferred to St. Joseph's Hospital where she had worked for 22 years. She was in therapy three times a day at St. Joseph's.

Mary Lou's left side had been affected. It took her four weeks to learn how to stand. She had more problems including headaches, but she persevered. Mary Lou was discharged after she learned how to walk up and down stairs.

When Mary Lou got home, she was unfocused. Christmas was coming, she felt disorganized, and her mind wasn't sharp at all. However, she now takes one step at a time, and it works. Mary Lou intentionally slows down because when she does things in a hurry she gets very frustrated.

She didn't understand the full impact of her stroke until she *did* return home. She decided to go ahead and do as much as possible- just as before, but within limits. Before her stroke Mary Lou was very independent. Now she depended on her husband for driving her to therapy, etc., but she accepted that.

Mary Lou's nature is to accept the way things are but be optimistic. Visits from her son, daughter, and two grandchildren help her remain optimistic. At one point, though Mary Lou didn't think she was depressed, she also didn't feel like eating. Her doctor thought she needed help, so brought in a psychologist to counsel her. He got her eating again.

Mary Lou's husband has played a key role in her recovery. He always pushes her to do what she should do. She's also disciplined. She sustains her recovery by attending every one of her therapy sessions. Mary Lou has even been complimented by her therapist for her disciplined approach.

In the early stages of her recovery she became very emotional, but eventually got over it. She finally reached the acceptance stage. Her attitude is to keep positive. Otherwise, she wouldn't make it.

Mary Lou's life focus hasn't essentially changed, although a new element has been added. Although her family and children's families are still important to her, she also wants to help other stroke survivors.

- *How long did it take you to face the reality of your situation? What helped you get to that stage?*
- *What did you learn from Mary Lou's story?*

As a survivor, facing reality also means getting as much information as possible about your condition. You 'own' that information. You have every legal right to obtain any medical records kept on you- CT scans, functional MRIs, etc. Getting all that information helps you to make better decisions about your future.

Summary Point

- **Realistic stroke survivors (eventually) accept their reduced competence but will not accept their inability to do something about it.**

Motivated and Optimistic

"I still find each day too short for all the thoughts I want to think, all the walks I want to take, all the books I want to read, and all the friends I want to see."
(John Burroughs)

Guiding Question:

What keeps you going?

Strong stroke survivors expect to increase their ability. In this way, they remain **motivated and optimistic**. They also understand that many stroke survivors are in worse condition than they are and that some who had a stroke died immediately.

Therefore, they consider themselves blessed. They're alive and they have a chance to improve. Their caregiver, moreover, often plays a key role in helping them remain motivated and optimistic. The lucky ones have good caregivers.

* *How motivated and optimistic are you? What motivates you?*

Zenta's Story

Zenta goes forward. She doesn't look back. She now has a greater appreciation of life and doesn't take anything for granted. Zenta always tries to be thankful. Since her stroke she sees her life as more enriched because of the people "who have been put in her life, particularly her husband, Jack (her caregiver) and best friend."

One morning Zenta woke to find her fingertips had gone numb. But that went away. Then from her head to her feet something felt strange. Jack took her to the hospital in Taunton, MA.

Zenta's husband thought she had had a heart attack.

When she was placed in a wheelchair, she had a stroke in the emergency room. After spending six days in a Boston ICU, she returned to Taunton, MA for six weeks of rehab.

When Zenta had her stroke she knew she was in deep trouble. She couldn't speak, hear, or see. Her whole left side was weak and her mouth drooped. However, six weeks of therapy not only improved the droop, but Zenta could now speak. She still wasn't able to walk.

Zenta's stroke took place six years ago. Her recovery has been remarkable, though she still has trouble with fine motor skills in her left hand. She has been very disciplined in her therapy and did everything the therapist asked her to do. Zenta now goes to the gym three times a week.

She feels that maintaining a good attitude is key to a good recovery. In going forward there's no time to be depressed. She's not going to let her stroke hold her back from enjoying life.

Zenta's new life focus of going forward, being thankful for what life has to offer, and not taking anything for granted has been anchored by her faith: "The joy of the Lord is my strength. Keep me going, Lord."

- *What kept Zenta moving forward?*
- *What keeps you moving forward? What keeps you optimistic and motivated?*

It's hard to keep optimistic and motivated when things get particularly difficult and painful. That's when you need to take a break and do something completely different. Or talk with your caregiver or physician. Or meditate and pray. Or count your blessings.

Greg's Story

Greg's stroke originated from strange timing and an even stranger cause.

Greg Ward had just been made partner in an international shipping company three months before his stroke. He had trouble with snoring so he decided to take an over-the-counter medication to address it. It was found out later that only three of the people who reacted to this medication actually survived. Thousands had died.

Anyway, Greg took one pill. The next morning his fiancé tried to wake him and couldn't. An ambulance was called to take him to the hospital. He still couldn't be wakened. They tested him for high blood pressure. Then he had a stroke.

Greg 'died,' but was resuscitated after he saw light in a tunnel. A month later he regained consciousness and found out he was paralyzed on the right side. Moreover, he could neither see nor hear on that side. When he walked like a drunkard, they tied him to his bed.

Greg slowly tried to improve, but was confused in the early days of his stroke. He wasn't able to reflect or analyze, so decisions were made for him. His family supported him until he returned to Florida to stay with his mother. He now lives on his own in Clermont, Florida, twenty miles west of Orlando.

Greg had to relearn how to read and write and now reads a chapter of the Bible every morning. Through this reading and watching sermons every week, "the Lord provides guideposts for him." Mornings work well. He reads the newspaper and is able to think. People visit him and provide communion. Greg is making the best of life that he can by dealing with who he is now.

Greg uses a three-wheeler bike to take an eleven

mile hilly road to Church and has got his time down to well below an hour. One of his joys is to wheel up to a nearby winery to listen to one of the outside musical concerts they sponsor.

He's always been motivated and never depressed. Although he still has facial and right side pain, he can deal with it. Meanwhile, his whole right side is getting stronger.

Greg focuses on getting better and is very disciplined. He writes everything down on the calendar and follows a schedule. He makes a list (including groceries) for almost everything he needs to do and sticks it in his notebook.

Greg feels that his family didn't get 'stuck' with him, so if he needs help he can ask for it. He can't do mechanical things with his right hand, so asks his brother to help him- such as fixing the sink. For the time being, Greg accepts his inability to do these things, but he doesn't give up. He's not impatient.

Before Greg had a stroke, his life was completely different. He had a lot of friends, had just become a partner in his firm, and was planning to get married. After the stroke, he wasn't able to work and his fiancé 'gave him back to his family.'

His helpful phrases? "Deal with who you are. Patience is a virtue. A smile always helps."

- *What part of your story is similar to Greg's?*
- *What 'helpful phrases' keep you going?*

There is no magic answer here. Part of what keeps us going simply comes from our character or nature. A good caregiver and good friends also make a big difference.

Have you noticed the difference in people's response to you when you greet them in a positive, optimistic way? Keep doing it. They benefit. So do you.

Summary Points

- **Keep moving forward.**
- **You're blessed. Act on it.**

Focused and Disciplined

"*Nothing will work unless you do.*"

Guiding Question:

How will you really improve your capability?

Because most stroke survivors have to deal with a range of disabilities, it's difficult to focus on the few that are really important. They're torn one way or another by spontaneous distractions.

Does this seem familiar? You start to do one particular thing like putting on your hat and coat to go on a doctor's appointment. But when you put on your hat, you realize you've left the dog outside, so you go get the dog.

As you're getting the dog, you see a piece of garbage on the ground which somebody had carelessly thrown out their car window. How could they do that? You pick up the garbage and put it in the garbage can.

Then you get into your car and suddenly realize you forgot to put your coat on. How in the world did I forget that?

I'm sure this never happens to you. Right?

- *How do you get distracted?*

What helps me on occasion is to think about the number of things I need to do before I take on another task. I focus on the number. That helps me to remember what those things are: 1. put on my hat. 2. Put on my coat. 3. Get the dog (forget the garbage for now). Three things. Three things. Now, what are they?

Putting lists together also helps, especially a 'To Do' list. Just remember where you put it.

Another type of distraction is based on not setting priorities. Do I work on buttoning my shirt buttons or pulling up my underwear and pants after going to the bathroom?

Buttoning my shirt buttons becomes important when I'm quickly preparing for a doctor's appointment. Pulling up my underwear/pants is crucial after going to the bathroom. I certainly don't want anybody else doing it for me if I can avoid it. So what's really more important to my confidence and well being?

In my mind, both are key everyday living skills. What should I concentrate on? More importantly, what should I practice? I can't decide, and will probably never learn to do either one very well- unless I practice.

- **What everyday thing do you need to focus on and practice?**

Chuck's Story

Now, here's a guy whose life was full before his stroke, but...

Chuck Hofvander, 56, who was a senior project manager for Xerox, had a young family and kept vigorously active. Now his life is full again, but in a radically different way. What happened? Read on...

Chuck had been healthy and rode a bike an average of 2,500 miles a year. When he wasn't riding, he ran and lifted weights. In 2004, Chuck had a hemorrhagic stroke while riding a stationary bike in his basement.

> *"I began feeling light headed. I came upstairs to the kitchen and my feeling of light headedness worsened. When it got to the point that I thought I would pass out, I went into our family room and that's where my wife found me two and a half hours later. The whole process lasted under five minutes. When you're alone, having a stroke, calling 911 doesn't come to mind.*

> *"When I was brought into the Northwest Comm. ER, the doctor gave my life no hope. The priest in attendance administered last rights. The neurosurgeon said, if she didn't operate in the next 15 minutes I would be gone. The neurosurgeon could not even guarantee that even if she did*

operate, that I wouldn't be in a coma for
the rest of my life or die on the table.

"I am adapting my 'new life.' I've come to
realize that after the stroke I wasted time
regretting my 'old life' and feeling sorry
for myself. The grieving and letting go of
my old life as I knew it was necessary.
It took over three years and with the help
of friends and family I finally realized it's
not a onetime process. It's an ongoing
process that never ends."

(from Chuck's writing)

Amazingly, through discussions with his wife, they discovered he was meant to have a stroke and bring hope to other stroke survivors.

So what does Chuck do now? He exercises, he enjoys his wife, children, and friends, and is involved with an aphasia club. The aphasia club meets once a week at their home. Besides giving speeches, Chuck attends these kinds of aphasia meetings up to three times a week. He finds it all very satisfying.

Chuck is extremely disciplined, and feels that self-determination is a key. He gets up every morning with a plan and determined to do the plan. The plan might include the act of getting up itself, making breakfast, doing the dishes, doing e-mail, and writing.

Chuck once worked at Combined Insurance of America. The renowned W. Clements Stone headed up the company. Stone continually used a phrase that inspired and continues to inspire Chuck: "I feel happy, healthy, and terrific."

- ***What is there in Chuck's story that 'resonates' with you?***
- ***How did Chuck stay focused and disciplined?***

Strong Stroke Survivors clearly know what competencies and skills will make a real difference in their lives. They are **focused and disciplined**. They likely have a sequence of learning targets. "I want to learn how to pull up my pants first. I'll worry about buttons later." Each time they go to the bathroom, they 'practice' pulling up their pants- trying one way or another until they've mastered the technique without consciously thinking about it.

For so-called 'normal' people it's hard to understand how somebody could forget how to pull up their underwear and pants. It's the same for stroke survivors. It becomes extremely frustrating because they used to know how to do it, but can't remember how they actually did do it. They're starting all over again. They sometimes feel like a child, but they also need to get on with their learning.

- **Overall, how do you build focus and discipline into your recovery?**

For strong stroke survivors, discipline is practiced in two different ways. Both are difficult. The first is intentionally to use their weak side to improve it. It is so much easier and quicker to use the strong side. All that does is further weaken the weak side.

Edward Taub, a breakthrough brain researcher, called this phenomenon 'learned non-use.' That part of the brain actually starts to weaken and is replaced by another part of the brain that is more actively used. 'Use it to improve it.'

- *How do <u>you</u> develop your 'weak side?'*

Secondly, is the issue of staying with your practice. When tired or cranky, it's tempting to let your practice go. Again, it's easy to take the simple way out- and not practice. It's less tiring and irritating.

However, Strong Stroke Survivors stay with it. That's not to say they don't have either forgetful or weak moments, but overall, they stay focused enough to cultivate even small improvements.

Other people may never notice any difference, but the strong ones take pride in their efforts and results. They also realize that without focus and discipline, they never would have improved. They continually test themselves to attain a higher level of competence.

- *Have you tested your capability limits recently? If so, how did you apply focus and discipline to improve your capability? If not, how could you apply focus and discipline now?*

Tony's Story

Tony Kenter, 50, lives in Mooresville, NC ('Race City'). He uses his hands for work. He's been a racing car driver, master mechanic, and now, crew chief. In truth, he needs more than his hands. He needs his whole body. And brain. But one day something gave way.

The day before Thanksgiving, it felt as if his legs had fallen asleep, but that sensation soon disappeared. The next morning, his left leg and arm went numb, so Tony went to the hospital to find out what was wrong. His blood pressure was slightly elevated, then highly elevated. They also found one little spot in his brain. He stayed in the hospital for five days. Tony had had a stroke.

Tony eventually regained most of his physical capability- he estimates about 95%. It took him only three months. He got rid of his cane, then his leg brace.

So, how did Tony do it?

Tony faced a daunting challenge. He had to get back to work as soon as possible. He had a wife and two children to support. He couldn't let them down.

Tony did all he could and more to regain his capability. However, he didn't know what his top limit was. He didn't worry about it. He just got to work- on his therapy. His long life in sports probably helped. You win a few. You lose a few. But you just keep going- and try as hard as possible.

Tony had the right attitude. He looked forward to therapy and considered it a challenge. Moreover, he enjoyed working with therapists and some of the other stroke patients.

Tony quickly began to see results from his hard work. He also noticed a number of older people who didn't want to be in therapy; they wanted to go home and do nothing. Tony didn't want go home and do nothing. Instead, he wanted to get back to 'normal' as soon as he could. Everyone told him he had a good chance.

Tony set goals for himself. He wanted to go down to Daytona at the end of January to test cars. His goal was to go there without a cane or brace. And so he did.

According to Tony, his major obstacle was not getting ahead as fast as he could. He reported in to his physician every couple of weeks, but felt he didn't get enough information from his neurologist. For Tony, feedback was important. After all, he wanted to know how he was doing in relation to the goals he had set for himself.

Tony was self-disciplined. Between visits to the clinic, he continually worked on his therapy at home. He followed up on all suggestions he got from his therapists.

There was something else. Tony tried to do everything

with his weak hand- picking up things, putting on clothes, working a wrench, etc. He also practiced standing in the doorway on his weak leg. These very processes Tony initiated on his own, paralleled new kinds of constraint induced therapy (CIT) neuroscientists like Edward Taub had pioneered. But Tony had never heard of CIT. He just thought it was a good idea. He feels that **had** he heard of CIT, he might have recovered more quickly.

Tony's resilience- his ability to bounce back from inevitable setbacks- was based, in part, on the support he received from both his family and employer. His employer was very flexible and supportive. Tony was under no pressure, and it was up to him how much work he did. The owner was willing to work with him in any way that was helpful.

Tony returned to full time work as shop manager in a few months.

- *How does Tony's story compare with your own?*
- *How did Tony practice focus and discipline?*

Of all the strong survivor characteristics, this one, focus and discipline, is the hardest to cultivate and carry out. It runs contrary to many of the situations most stroke survivors face: low energy, fractured view of things, easily distracted, difficulty remembering anything, emotional upheavals, etc.

However, without focus and discipline, it's unlikely you'll be successful in improving your capability. So work on it!

Summary Points

- **Do the difficult thing: use your weak side**
  - **Use numbers and lists**
  - **Practice, practice, practice!**

Purposeful and Determined

"It's the constant and determined effort that breaks down all resistance, sweeps away all obstacles."

(Claude M. Bristol)

Guiding Question:

How do your life purpose and determination 'anchor' you in your recovery?

Strong stroke survivors also demonstrate clear purpose. They know why they're alive. Maybe they haven't figured out why they in particular survived such a devastating personal event, but they're not hesitant to move forward.

A strong **purpose** and **determination** are significant factors in keeping them going.

Gert's Story

Gert's story is essentially a Gert and Kara story. Kara is Gert's wife, caregiver, advocate, and coach. For our purposes now, however, we're going to cover just Gert's side of the story. Gert had his stroke about eight months after he and Kara got married.

But let's start at the beginning... Gert Roosen,

38, lives in Silver Spring, Maryland. In 2005 Gert started seeing double, so he talked to a couple of doctors. They discovered a tumor and put him on steroids. He was worried because his sister had had a brain tumor while in her teens. His tumor was subsequently removed six weeks after they discovered it. It was benign. Gert felt lucky because he was working with a good neurologist and receiving the best of care at Johns Hopkins.

Two weeks after his brain operation, Gert was on the way to rehab and didn't feel well. He suffered a stroke, a hemorrhagic stroke.

He now walks with a cane. Although he knows he's strong, he lacks confidence because he's not sure where his leg is. He lacks positional awareness because he can't see his right leg. Once in a while he experiences pain in his face.

What keeps Gert going is his determination to do everything necessary to get well. His wife, Kara, and his good friends stand by him. In looking back, Gert feels his medical problems were the best thing that ever happened to him.

As Gert continues his recovery, he feels essentially motivated, though slips once in a while. He's fairly disciplined but only because he has to be- if he wants to improve. His main driving focus is to get well. He is sustained by his stubbornness and good therapy.

Gert's view of things? "Never give up. Look on the bright side of things. It happened. So what? Move on."

- ***What 'fuels' Gert's moving forward?***
- ***What fuels your moving forward?***

Your view of the world probably changed after your stroke. More than likely, you asked yourself a lot of serious questions- some of which you could answer, some you couldn't. Did any of those questions include why you were spared, why you were still alive? If so, answering that question likely clarified your life purpose.

However, your life purpose may not have changed. Or it might have changed a little or a lot (I'm in the latter group). Regardless, one way or another, it's likely a clearer purpose. That clearer purpose alone will fuel your determination to fulfill it.

Whew! Heavy stuff, but important stuff for a stroke survivor, because that determination to fulfill your life purpose will pull you forward, get you unstuck.

- ***What do you see as your life purpose?***
- ***How determined are you to fulfill that purpose? What makes you that determined?***

Patrice's Story

Patrice didn't have any of the normal stroke warnings. One day her hand simply twitched on the patio door. The next morning she couldn't use the left side of her body.

Patrice lived in an area of no phones. She also had no car and lived half a mile from the nearest road, so she walked up to the road and called for help. She remembers nothing of her climb- only the deer at the top of the road. After a couple of trucks passed by, she walked into the middle of the road to stop the next truck. The driver took her to her brother's home; then her brother took her to the hospital.

Patrice didn't know if she had had a stroke, but the hospital confirmed it the next day. They also told her she wouldn't be able to use her left hand. They offered to send her to rehab, but she didn't want to go (she had been a rehab nurse). After five days, Patrice went home.

She couldn't dress, cook, or do anything. Although a nurse visited her three times, Patrice decided to use holistic medicine to heal herself. She knew enough about rehab, so she trained herself. Eventually she was able to get her hand to move.

Patrice knew her second stroke *was* a stroke. She did call her doctor, but told him she wasn't going to the hospital. The doctor insisted on her going even though she didn't have any insurance or money.

After her second stroke, angioplasty was performed on her neck. They gave her a 40% chance of coming off the table. At that point, she "gave it all away," and *did* come off the table. She also felt her stubbornness made a difference.

Surprisingly, Patrice feels that the third stroke rewired her brain! She can think more clearly now. However, her thinking is more black and white. She cautions others not to ask her anything if they don't want an honest answer.

Although she has a little numbness now, it took four years to rehabilitate herself to this point. During that period she had two more strokes, one of them hemorrhagic. As a result, there have been a number of residual effects; at times, she can move only two fingers.

Although she decided to live with her disability, she was not going to give up the fight. "When people give in, that's it. As long as you have fight in you, you can make it." Moreover, Patrice didn't want to be a burden either to her kids or roommate nor did she want to live in a nursing home. "If I wanted 'quality of life' I had to fight for it."

Patrice is very religious. She "turned a lot of stuff over to God." When she couldn't concentrate enough to watch TV, read a book, or do any crafts, she talked to God.

Patrice forced herself to do things that were difficult. For example, she fed 'her' deer three times a day. They took food out of her hand, but she had to brace the bag in her left hand. It was hard. Moreover, the deer would get impatient. However, it kept her going. Patrice felt if she didn't feed the deer, they wouldn't make it. And she probably wouldn't make it either. The deer saved her.

Over time, Patrice has become more determined to do 'whatever' to the best of her ability. Moreover, she says, "Life is short. You don't know what's going to happen. Enjoy it while you can. There's an old adage: 'A man is feeling sorry for himself because he has no shoes to put on his feet. Then he meets a man who has no feet.' Somebody is worse off, so deal with it."

- *What kept Patrice going?*
- *What did you learn from her story that will help you?*

For stroke survivors, purpose and determination come from many places: shock, anger, reflection. For some, it's a simple matter- to survive day to day. Whatever it is, it fuels your moving ahead. Treasure it.

Summary Points

- **Clarify your purpose**
- **Fill up your tank with 'fuel'**
- **Go forward!**

Resilient

"Man never made any material as resilient as the human spirit."

(Bern Williams)

Guiding Question:

How do you overcome inevitable difficulties and obstacles in your recovery?

Almost all stroke survivors experience moments of weakness and self-doubt. However, their personal reasons for living and their will to carry on the best way they can, sustains them through these trying periods.

- *What continues to sustain you through your difficult periods?*

These special survivors show **resilience**. That is, when faced with inevitable obstacles and setbacks, they're able to bounce back. Some survivors can come back from an extended series of challenging setbacks and simply keep going. They don't seem to get frustrated with all the 'commotion.' Their course is clear: straight ahead.

Stroke is a complex condition. It can be manifested in so many ways and accompanied by a unique set of disabilities. For some people, their disabilities can be relatively easy to overcome. Others face what seem to be insurmountable obstacles. It's this latter group in particular who have to be truly resilient in order to survive.

- *How have you demonstrated resilience in your recovery?*

Jim's Story

When Jim, 61, suffered an ischemic stroke four years ago, he was confused because his brain wasn't working properly. He couldn't even remember the 911 number. Finally his neighbors gave him a ride to the hospital where he spent ten days in recovery. Then his cousin, who was married to a nurse, arranged for him to go to a rehab hospital in Alexandria, VA.

One year after Jim's stroke, he was receiving therapy and told the therapist his legs didn't feel good. So Jim went to his doctor and found out he had had a second stroke (a TIA). The doctor put him on medication.

Communication was virtually impossible. He couldn't read, write or speak. However, he became particularly disciplined in his speech drills and is currently working on his reading and writing.

Jim has difficulty reading more than five pages at a time. He can't spell, and it takes him more than an hour to write three lines. When he sends emails at work, he is short and sweet. Jim now works in communication systems for the Department of Defense.

What's kept Jim going? He responds, "Why not? Life is full of setbacks. You're born, you pay taxes, you die." How has his life changed? "I appreciate life more and help other people. Before my stroke, I was a loner. Now I have a lot of supportive friends. I need them. They make an important difference in my life."

Final comments? "The brain is a wonderful organ. Based on the theory of neuroplasticity, it is possible to train your brain. But it takes a long time to develop new pathways. Every stroke is different. You have to deal with it by zeroing in on your problems and get therapy. Train your brain."

Jim's father died of a stroke, so at this point, Jim feels lucky to be alive- and able to pay for his recovery. Jim's whole life now is recovery. His sole motivation is to get better.

- *Like Jim, how have you 'trained your brain?'*

Certain survivors draw from some inner life force that 'steels' them for the battles ahead. They're able to take on tough challenges and respond positively to them. Those with extreme disabilities obviously are tested the most.

In some cases, their daunting impediments stimulate creative solutions. One survivor uses a three-wheeled bike to haul his dog around in a cart behind him. He clearly models both resilience and creativity.

Susan's Story

Susan suffered a stroke at the age of nine. She was playing a new game with her brother and a few friends at the kitchen table. It's the last thing she remembers.

After two weeks in the hospital, Susan spent the following four months in physical therapy. She celebrated her tenth birthday in the hospital. In a picture of herself with her mother and a new friend, her right eye and mouth are turned down, but she is still smiling.

During her four months in therapy at Holy Cross in Detroit, Susan learned the basics of how to walk, how to talk, and how to move the fingers on her right hand. Her mother followed the doctor's instructions and very quickly sent her back to school where classmates helped her button and unbutton her coat and carry her books. Teachers taped papers to her desk so she could learn to write again. She survived those four months, but never wishes to repeat it.

Susan has gone through therapy six different times. After a near-accident with her first child, she undertook three months of occupational therapy at a clinic where, for the first time, they helped her right hand and arm dexterity. She was also treated for aphasia. Susan feels that "these therapists in Colorado worked my mind and body and I will forever be in their debt."

After moving to Maryland to start a new life for

herself, Susan had to be treated at the National Rehabilitation Hospital three times- for her right foot, Achilles tendon, and right knee. She's had therapy off and on most of her life. According to Susan, "the first time you go in to see a therapist, you will come out hurting more than when you went in. But in the long run, they help tremendously."

Since gaining a Master of Science degree from the University of Maryland, Susan has worked as a senior engineer on a Federal Aviation Administration contract at ITT Industries. Recently she and another stroke survivor launched a new non-profit organization to assist the disabled- Circle of Rights, Inc. In her view, she has done more than survive. Susan has become a productive member of society.

- *What did you learn about yourself from Susan's story?*
- *How can you personally apply what you have learned from Susan's story?*

Resilience obviously comes from inside and has something to do with genetics. However, there is much you can do to build your resilience. The most important is to keep in good health: eat right, sleep right, exercise right, etc. Resilience is almost a composite, an end product of all your other strengths.

One very direct way to build your resilience is to build your endurance. In the early going most of us have little energy to address even the simplest of tasks without getting worn out.

Here's an example. I wanted to build my wife a potting bench. And I didn't want to use any power tools; they were too dangerous. So I had to cut a number of 2X4s and 4X4s by hand.

At the start, all I could do was make *one cut a day-* then rest the remainder of the day. I knew I could do better, but I didn't know how to build my endurance- simply because most of the things I used to do were no longer available to me. Until I found water aerobics.

Although the classes were an hour long, initially I would climb out of the pool after only ten minutes. That was all I could do. I finally built it up to half an hour and seemed to get stuck. Then one day I broke through to a whole hour. I was really excited. I found it hard to believe.

Now I can stay up a whole day from 5:00 in the morning until 9:00 at night (5 to 9- not 9 to 5) without resting once. I can also cut an almost unlimited number of pieces of wood in a day- with only small pauses in between.

Build your resilience by building your endurance.

Summary Point

- **Draw on all your strengths to bounce back from inevitable setbacks- be resilient**

Mr. Pete's Story

Part 2

One time Mr. Pete's doctor met his wife in the parking lot while he was on the way home. She told him her concerns about her husband's well-being. The doctor decided to come back to Mr. Pete's hospital bed to tell him, "There's always hope." It eventually became part of the name of Mr. Pete's recovery organization.

Mr. Pete obviously demonstrated remarkable will in his lengthy recovery (over a period of three years). However, he claims he could never have done it alone. The support of wife and family were critical to his survival. Despite that support, he still went through bouts of depression he didn't even recognize at the time.

In considering his future, Mr. Pete realized two things. It wouldn't be like his former life, and he didn't want it to be like his former life. He had spent too much energy getting things and keeping people from getting in his way.

Now he wanted to help people help themselves— particularly stroke survivors. Eventually he formed an organization, Hope for Stroke (hope4stroke. com, 1-888-229-4616 toll-free), to fulfill that new ambition.

Sharing his personal story at the bedside of recent

stroke survivors encouraged them to tell their stories and take the first few steps in their recovery.

Mr. Pete feels that although the brain is complicated, it's an easy thing to use. The brain needs to be challenged to take out its 'toolkit' to repair the part that's not working—that any traumatic injury to it can be addressed.

Hope for Stroke aligns brain with the body. Mr. Pete feels too many people get locked into their disbelief-that further improvement in their capability is not possible. However, he believes in the neuroplasticity of the brain. It's been the key to his overcoming so many obstacles, and may well be the key for others.

Mr. Pete's words of encouragement to others? "Don't give up. It's only another step in the marathon." *

* Mr. Pete should know. He ran four of them before his stroke.

Strong Stroke Survivors: A Summary

In summary, the following characteristics frame a few of the life forces of a strong stroke survivor. The author also asked a small sample of these people (the eleven people in the stories you read) to assess themselves in relation to the five characteristics. On a 5 point scale, 1 is Low and 5, High. Here are the results:

Strong Stroke Survivor Characteristics	SSS Ratings
Purposeful and Determined	4.9
Realistic	4.8
Motivated and Optimistic	4.8
Resilient	4.8
Focused and Disciplined	4.2

Purposeful/Determined came out the highest on this micro-survey, with **Realistic**, **Motivated/ Optimistic** and **Resilient** close behind. Even though this was a very small survey of eleven stroke survivors (which would not hold up statistically), overall these are extremely high scores. **Focused/ Disciplined** trailed the others but was still rated as a high characteristic at 4.2 out of 5.

Keep in mind these are self-ratings, not ratings by some more objective observer. On the other hand, in responding to this small survey, these admirable people rarely hesitated to provide a self-assessment. They knew who they were.

- *If you want to see how you stack up against these characteristics, use the same 5-point scale (1- Low; 5- High) to rate yourself. If your caregiver rates you as well, you'll really have something to talk about!*

- *Which characteristic is your strongest? Which is your 'weakest'? How could you improve?*

It's difficult to know whether these strong stroke survivors were as strong before their strokes as they are now. However, I suspect in a number of cases, their stroke actually strengthened them.

Summary Points

- **Here are the five Strong Stroke Survivor Characteristics (Remember them and practice them!):**
  - **Realistic**
  - **Motivated and optimistic**
  - **Focused and disciplined**
  - **Purposeful and determined**
  - **Resilient**

Third Section
POWERFUL CAREGIVERS

"Too often we underestimate the power of a smile, a kind word, a listening ear, an honest compliment, or the smallest act of caring, all of which have the potential to turn a life around."

(Leo Buscaglia)

Guiding Question:

How does a caregiver shift gears with the survivor so that each helps the other to grow?

Stroke caregivers are not usually trained in this role. They grow into it. As with stroke survivors themselves, some do better at it than others. Here's a rough sketch of the powerful caregiver roles that nicely complement that of the strong stroke survivor.

Caregiver Roles

In the early going, the powerful caregiver is probably unaware of the multiple roles he/she has undertaken: a) supporter; b) model; c) teacher/

learner. These are ongoing during the survivor recovery period.

The supporter role is an obvious one. However, a fine line has to be drawn here. The stroke survivor needs all the support he can get. He's climbing a steep, rock-strewn mountain. Slipping and falling back is common on the path to recovery. So is depression. Caregivers have to be ever watchful, particularly in the early going, to help the survivor get going.

However, too much support may lead to too much dependency. The stroke survivor has to be given every chance to try something on her own- obviously within appropriate safety constraints. Also, too much support may lead to too much control—by the caregiver—which can pose major problems later on.

- *As a stroke survivor, where are you on the road to independence? Choose a number ('1' is Not at All, '10' is totally Independent). What is one small step you could take toward more independence?*

- *As a caregiver, how have you acted as a model, learner, and teacher? Any specific examples?*

Whether the caregiver is aware of it or not, she acts as a model. Her behavior can be a powerful influence on the survivor who, in turn, may want to emulate her behavior. Don't forget. Caregivers also need caring—and time off. The stroke survivor can make it easier for the caregiver to take that time off without feeling guilty.

The caregiver also acts as both teacher and learner. The caregiver teacher's competence comes from her learning capability. As the stroke survivor becomes more independent- even if slightly- the caregiver has to make note of it so that she can figure out the next step to independence. That's called learning before teaching. In some instances, teaching simply means providing the survivor with more information on stroke recovery, support, and medications.

There's so much for the survivor to learn, relearn, and in some instances, unlearn. And the closest every-day person to facilitate that learning is the caregiver.

Caregiver 'Stages'

The fundamental stroke survivor caregiver role evolves through different stages and requires continuous adjustment as:

- Advocate
- Coach
- Coordinator

Obviously these roles are neither discrete nor necessarily sequential. They will overlap.

Advocate

Caregivers learn this role early and quickly. So many important decisions have to be made- and in a hurry. Caregivers feel pressured to make those decisions and take action before they are quite ready. As a result, the caregiver may lean too heavily on medical professionals for their expert guidance. However, they're not always 'right.' On occasion, caregivers must be prepared to challenge that expert advice on behalf of their survivors.

The advocate caregiver stands up for his or her survivor and asks tough questions at difficult times. After all, the survivor is barely surviving. A 'strong suggestion' or heated directive can make a huge difference.

It happened during my first few survival days- and it wasn't even my caregiver who did it. Just her best friend- right after I was 'coptered' for brain surgery to save my life.

Leaning way over the Neurology Admitting Desk when the neurologist was scanning my brain imaging documents, and in no uncertain terms, she delivered: "We didn't have Bob 'evacked' here for further analysis. He needs brain surgery now!"

Fingers immediately hit the telephone buttons, dialing the brain surgery team about 2:00 am. I was operated on that morning as the polls were opening for the 2004 presidential election (and there's more to that story).*

* My caregiver's best friend is now an outstanding child advocate in Texas.

- **How has your caregiver acted as an advocate for you?**

Coach

Coaching, of course, starts with safety- clearing pathways, putting up railings, and so on. Some things the survivor might have to learn on her own such as certain bathroom duties, etc. Other things such as 'transfers' the caregiver will have to coach her on.

Teaching is more direct than coaching. Coaching requires 'nudging.' In behavioral therapy, it's called shaping. If the caregiver coach can help the survivor take one small step toward the agreed-upon goal, it should be rewarded, even if it's a small reward.

It's difficult for the caregiver to know everything needed- both what to coach and how to coach. Likely the caregiver hasn't been in this position before- so there's lots of learning in the moment.

What's key is repetition and reward. The caregiver could rarely make a mistake by over-coaching. Moreover, the survivor fumbles and forgets. Both require caregiver patience.

- **What coaching/learning moment do you treasure as a survivor?**

Coordinator

The caregiver needs to coordinate so many things:

doctor and therapist visits, medication dispensing and refilling. Here again understanding and patience are mandatory. The stroke survivor is slow- both in physical coordination and thinking (but not in intelligence).

Unfortunately, the caregiver is running at a different pace- certainly much quicker. This difference in pacing can cause problems, resulting in frustration and sometimes aggravation for both parties.

That's when a sense of humor can save the day. 'Finding the funny' in a situation can provide a welcome relief from the intense relationship and mutual responsibility each has undertaken.

- ***What's a humorous moment that both you, as survivor, and your caregiver shared?***

Of course, the caregiver needs time on her own- to relax, enjoy, and recharge. That's when the stroke survivor needs to be patient, supportive and encouraging. Both 'need' each other, and when it's done right, the ever-changing relationship can be deeply satisfying.

- ***As a stroke survivor, what one thing could you do to help your caregiver 'survive?'***

CAREGIVER: FIVE PERSPECTIVES

'Getting Down To Basics' Caregiver: Betty, 75

The caregiver's role starts in the hospital. The number one issue is safety. Clear a path to things-particularly to the bathroom at night. Initially, you might have to have a commode by the bedside. Provide handles in the bathroom so the stroke survivor can grab 'em and hang onto 'em.

You might also need a safety belt for that wheelchair. Ensure the brakes are locked and foot pedals out of the way before you put your survivor in it. Make sure the weak hand is up so it doesn't get caught in the wheelchair. Survivors sometimes feel uncomfortable if somebody other than their caregiver is pushing their wheelchair. Be cautious.

Be sure tables and chairs are the right height. Make sure clothes are facing up before they're put on and put the belt on first. Use stretchy socks and elastic shoestrings. Use button hooks and sock aids.

Always ask for a sharp knife at the restaurant. Be sure to put his chair in front of something interesting. Be careful of heavy doors. Put your foot in first, wedge your body in backwards, then let the door push the survivor in (not recommended for those who are a little unstable).

Sometimes the caregiver needs to be in front to guide

the survivor in walking and climbing. When going downstairs, stay behind and hang onto his belt and the railing.

Use various systems and reminders for taking pills. Also watch out for *low* blood pressure. It causes dizziness.

The caregiver is the survivor's 'seeing eye dog.' However, ensure he does everything by himself- or until he becomes over-frustrated.

Always be aware of survivors' limitations. Always build confidence. Their intelligence is the same, but their emotions are somewhat different. Their personality changes.

Caregivers do need a relief.

Betty might know what she's talking about. Her dear husband, Max, has had five strokes.

'The Sparker' Caregiver: Gail

Gail and Bob were members of our stroke support group. Then they moved to another state. So in their new hometown, Hudson, Ohio, Gail started up a stroke support group which now has 19 members. No ordinary caregiver here. She's a 'sparker.'

Gail sees the caregiver's role as a big responsibility: to help the survivor become more independent. For example, 'conveniences' need to be provided so the survivor can do things for himself.

As a caregiver, Gail is a learner. She's learned so much from other stroke survivors and caregivers that she can apply to Bob's and her situation. Gail has also learned from reading. And from Bob himself. Bob suffers from 'reflex crying' that seems to be out of his control. Gail has learned to ask him, "Is this a happy crying or is there something wrong?"

Gail's counsel to a new caregiver? Accept help. Don't be too independent. Don't go it alone. You could end up doing a great disservice to your survivor-especially during the first six months.

Husband or wife survivors need to know they're loved intuitively and that they're the most important person in the caregiver's life. However, you can love too much. Let him do up his own buttons.

The Evolving Role of Caregiver: Kara, 39

Eight months after Kara married Gert he was operated on for a brain tumor which turned out to be benign. However, two weeks after the operation he had a stroke. So Kara learned early how to be a caregiver.

Gert was 4.5 months in the hospital and rehab before he came home. This is how Kara became an advocate. Kara had to check on the nurses carefully to ensure they did the right thing.

Kara's counsel to caregivers is "to watch nurses like a hawk." Kara felt the need to be present- and be 'hyper-vigilant.' She was always around. She was loud. And it made a difference.

Another message to caregivers: "Do not be intimidated. Do not take everything as the truth. Do not be mesmerized by statistics." She found doctors to be essentially negative. The best prognosis was couched as 'hopefully.' She knew different. So did Gert's neurologist. He had a better view of 'the big picture.'

As a caregiver, it's so easy to give up. Sometimes you feel overwhelmed by the medical profession. They talk about studies that have been conducted-many of which stop at the end of the first year after a stroke. What happens after that is largely dependent on the caregiver, not the medical profession.

So the most important characteristic of a caregiver is a sense of humor. You have to be able to laugh because everything is so intense.

Caregiver as Complement: Veronica

Realistic

The caregiver can play a key role in helping the stroke survivor understand what really happened. Any questions need to be met head on—just the facts. And it needs to be repeated over and over again. The survivor has a hard time remembering the details, but needs to fill in the gaps. Otherwise, the survivor lives with too much uncertainty and too many unanswered questions. The caregiver helps to build memory.

Repeating what actually happened helps the caregiver understand the learning a stroke survivor is going through. Moreover, the repetition helps caregivers nurture their own patience.

Motivated, Optimistic

The caregiver needs to be encouraging and not be consumed by self-pity. Equally important, the caregiver has to be watchful about directing any negativity or blame toward the survivor.

Small improvements, such as using a fork, need to be surfaced, recognized, and celebrated. As a model for the stroke survivor, the caregiver has to remain optimistic. It rubs off on the survivor. Each day has to be met with a smile.

Communication (just talking together) draws the survivor 'back into the world.' The survivor needs to be kept engaged.

Focused, Disciplined

Any routines that are in place need to be supported. Moreover, life has to be kept simple as possible. Clutter needs to be removed. 'Too much stuff', whether it's mental, emotional, social or physical distracts and upsets the survivor.

Purposeful, Determined

The key purpose of the caregiver/survivor relationship is to build the survivor's independence-as much as possible, and as difficult as it is, as soon as possible.

The purpose of survivors helping others (particularly other stroke survivors) starts the cycle of understanding their own situation as survivors.

Resilient

The caregiver needs to be more than encouraging. Deep conversations need to reinforce the survivor's strengths, their demonstrated willpower and their determined focus. The caregiver needs to ask questions of the survivor that reinforce personal strengths.

Resilience has to be nurtured.

'How Do I Look' Caregiver: Mary

Mary Hawkes was an outstanding caregiver for her father, Charles Memrick. Both were members of the local support group (Charles is still an active member). Mary died recently. However, she left behind a tremendous legacy that her sister, Julie, now builds on for her father.

Mary wrote a piece for caregivers. It grew out of a special moment she and her father shared. It was handed out to our stroke support group. Indirectly, it's a wonderful tribute to Mary and the kind of gracious care she provided her father. Here it is.

Help Me- Help You
Caregiver 101

I believe that My Dad, Charles Memrick and I, Mary Hawkes have greatly benefited from the Stroke Survivor Support Group.

In an effort to give back to the group I would like to make an observation that my Dad has taught me recently that has greatly improved (I feel) my approach as a Caregiver.

Dad has been asking me before leaving for out-patient therapy, doctor's appointments, for a family visit, or when completing a meal out **"How do I look?"** *What a simple but reflective question that I feel gives me permission as the Caregiver to check and comb his hair, wipe his face, and clean his beard, gently recommend he change his shirt if it is stained and recommend suitable clothing for the intended trip. It establishes loving boundaries between my Dad as Stroke Survivor and me the daughter as Caregiver. It also allows me to let Dad continue to improve in his hygiene and his own personal care without my comments on his appearance upsetting him or demoralizing him. I don't have to wonder if I've offended him in helping*

him with daily activities and I know he cares how he looks and how others see him. This is a normal stage of recovery when we have the strength and desire to become the best we can become.

Now that my Dad had his first cataract removed I am looking forward to even greater improvement in his daily activities as he will now be able to see better and get back to his writing and other activities that were hampered by bad eyesight.

As the question of how to improve the interaction between stroke-survivor and caregiver continues to come up I hope this small communication tip helps. Thank you.

Mary Hawkes

The Caregiver's Role in the RAISE Program

The three week RAISE program in the following section works best if a powerful caregiver collaborates with the survivor. Caregiving, at this point, could even involve a whole team of caregivers.

The most important role and responsibility? Caring, coaching and believing that the survivor can improve her capability through the program.

The caregiver **coordinates the program as follows**:

1. Reviews the whole RAISE program with the survivor

1. Helps the survivor determine the specific capability to be worked on by reviewing the first three steps of RAISE: **Reflect, Analyze, and Identify**

1. Conducts the **Preliminary Assessment**, and determines with the survivor whether he/she is ready to proceed (How badly does the survivor want it?)

1. With the survivor, completes the three week **Capability Improvement Plan (Start):**

   - Helps to establish goals, measures, and exercises—they need to be stretch goals, but **SAFE** goals and exercises

   - Thinks creatively in discussing and establishing these key dimensions of the program

   - Discusses and agrees about how much time will be devoted to the program each day (suggested format is three practice rounds of each exercise each morning and afternoon/evening- and one practice session- three rounds- on each Saturday and Sunday)

- Conducts the **Initial Assessment** to determine baseline data from which progress will be measured

- At the end of each week, the caregiver reviews: a) how the survivor has progressed; b) whether or not he/she has kept up with the exercises; c) what changes might need to be made and d) what plans are for the following week

- Upon conclusion of the three-week program, the caregiver conducts, with the survivor, a **Final Assessment** of her capability (the assessment has to include the identical measures used in the Initial Assessment)

- Completes, with the caregiver the program pages that reveal the percentage improvement (or otherwise) in the survivor's specific capability

- Reviews the results with the survivor, discussing what worked, what didn't work, and why

- Celebrates, with the survivor, the survivor's disciplined effort and encouraging results

- Reviews with the survivor how to maintain or even increase the hard-won capability improvement

- Considers next steps which might mean starting a new RAISE program focused on a different specific capability

The RAISE program draws on all the caregiver's strengths and roles: model, learner, and teacher; advocate, coach and coordinator.

The caregiver 'models' the optimism and determination the survivor needs, to stay with the program to completion. By observing the survivor struggle through the early rounds of practice, the caregiver learns how to make any necessary changes to the program. The caregiver, as 'teacher,' guides the survivor through the RAISE process.

Advocacy comes into play when the caregiver and survivor 'ask' their physician, neurologist or therapist to approve the RAISE program. The caregiver as coach is put into practice in the feedback sessions with the survivor. "How do you think you're doing so far? What isn't working? How can we make the practice sessions work better for you?" etc. As coordinator, the caregiver reminds the survivor of the goals, practice sessions, and measurements, and reinforces the need to carry through with them.

Obviously the RAISE process not only challenges the survivor, but challenges the caregiver as well. All dimensions of the role need to be called into play for the RAISE program to work. Caregiver is a key to the door of rebuilding capability.

Summary Points

- **The caregiver continually draws on his/her strengths as model, learner and teacher**
- **The caregiver, in relation to survivor, 'grows' through the stages of advocate, coach and coordinator**
- **The caregiver acts as a key to the success of the RAISE program because the caregiver CARES**

Fourth Section
REBUILDING CAPABILITY (RAISE)

"A heart to resolve, a head to contrive, and a hand to execute."

(Edward Gibbon)

Guiding Question:

How can I improve one specific capability?

You've been on an unbelievable journey- unlike anybody else's. Now we're going to help you take your next constructive step on that journey. We're going to help you rebuild your capability. Probably not all of it. That may not be possible. But your taking one small step might indeed be possible. And we won't really know until we try.

First of all:

CAUTIONARY NOTE

Don't try anything until you've had your physician's approval, neurologist's approval or at least your therapist's approval. WE'RE NOT TAKING ANY RISKS TO YOUR HEALTH OR WELL-BEING.

Instead, we're going to lift you up- we're going to **RAISE** you- no, not literally or magically lift you into the air. Rather, we're going to raise your capability. You'll have to be focused and committed. So this is a further cautionary note:

It ain't gonna be easy!

Here's what's going to be easy: we'll provide a form you can take to your physician, neurologist or therapist so that he or she can better understand what you're up to- **that you're undertaking a small exercise to improve a specific capability.**

As you might recall, **RAISE** means **'rouse, restore to life'** (The Concise Oxford Dictionary). This definition will now act as our guide, our vision as we go forward.

The following sub-sections will take you, step-by-step through the RAISE process to improve a specific ability. These steps correspond to the **RAISE** letters. Surprise, surprise!

Your caregiver (and coach) will help you understand and complete the first three steps (**R**eflect, **A**nalyze, **I**dentify). Then, with your caregiver, you plan for improvement and carry out your plan (**S**tart). Finally, your caregiver and you will see how you've done. (**E**valuate).

- **Step 1: R—Reflect**
- **Step 2: A—Analyze**
- **Step 3: I—Identify**
- **Step 4: S—Start**
- **Step 5: E—Evaluate**

Another thing, this particular exercise **has not** been tried on hundreds of people- only a few stroke survivors (including myself). However, so far it has worked for all those who stuck with the program. We've each achieved results beyond our expectations.

But it may not work for you. The key is the *right attitude*. Remember all the strong stroke survivor stories you read? *They* had the right attitude. *They* were **motivated**.

Strong motivation is the key to RAISE success. We've even designed a self-assessment (the Preliminary Assessment) to 'test' how strongly you want to improve your capability. If you really aren't 'there' yet, then I suggest you work on something else to get you motivated..

Enough. Let's get started.

Introduction

Before you, the survivor, start the RAISE program, 'test' your readiness to undertake it by completing the following assessment:

Preliminary Assessment

1. What keeps you going from day to day?

2. How much do you think you could increase a specific capability?
   - 1- 0%
   - 2- 25%
   - 3- 50%
   - 4- 75%
   - 5- 100%

3. What will motivate you to increase it?

4. If you do increase a specific capability, how will that help you?

5. If you don't increase your capability during the exercises, will you still be motivated to improve? Why?

6. In the past, when you undertook a plan to improve yourself, how well did you 'stick with it?'

   - Not at all
   - Minimally
   - Moderately
   - Strongly
   - Totally

7. What is the biggest hurdle you have to overcome in carrying out a plan?

8. What helps you stay with a plan?

9. What makes you 'ready' now to undertake the RAISE program?

10. How committed are you to carrying out the RAISE program?

   - Not committed at all
   - Minimally committed
   - Moderately committed
   - Very committed
   - Totally committed

11. To what degree can you focus on a goal or objective?

   - Not focused at all
   - Easily distracted
   - Moderately focused
   - Occasionally distracted
   - Totally focused

12. How long can you stay with a task you want to do?

   - 5 minutes
   - 10 minutes
   - 20 minutes
   - 30 minutes
   - An hour or more

13. How much 'mind garbage' gets in your way?

    - A lot
    - Frequently gets in the way
    - Moderate amount
    - Rarely have to deal with it
    - Totally clear mind

14. How do you deal with it?

15. What makes you a good candidate for the RAISE program?

The Caregiver's Role: RAISE Overview

First of all, the caregiver has to stimulate the survivor to start the RAISE program. Gettin' goin' is clearly the first step. Initial motivation shouldn't be difficult because this total exercise focuses on the survivor increasing some specific capability. Only those survivors who have truly given up on themselves would be reluctant to take the first step.

So how does the caregiver get the survivor goin'? By reminding her of the new research that shows no matter when the stroke occurred or what the survivor's age is, the brain is still capable of learning and changing. Certain changes may be extremely difficult, and perhaps impossible. Others will come much more easily.

However, nobody really knows which is which—including the survivor. There's only one way of finding out—and that's to try it. This is the time to gently persuade your survivor that there's very little to lose and much to gain by giving RAISE a try. However, the survivor does have to be truly motivated to improve her capability even in some small way. Otherwise, the program will not work.

In one sense, the caregiver acts as an advocate for the survivor by encouraging her to try the RAISE program because it's in the best interests of the survivor.

Step 1: Reflect (RAISE)

"As human beings, we have the privilege to make our thoughts more real than anything else, and when we do, the brain records those impressions in the deep folds of its tissues. Mastering this skill allows us to begin to rewire our brains..."

(Joe Dispenza, Evolve Your Brain)

Guiding Questions:

What personal strengths can you draw on to continue your recovery?

What increased capability would make the biggest difference to you? Why?

In the initial stages of stroke recovery, it's difficult to understand exactly what happened to you. Your brain is a thick fog. You are muddled and confused.

- *What was your brain like right after your stroke?*

At some point, things start to clear a little. You *do* begin to understand what happened to you. More importantly, you realize two contradictory things: you feel blessed because you're still alive but devastated by your condition and the consequences that flow from it.

- *How did you clarify what was going on?*

So the journey—and struggle—begin. So many issues have to be addressed, and seemingly all at once. Right after the crisis, health issues are mixed in with other critical arrangements that need to be made. However, we know your route back to health is more important than anything else. And that journey to better health and increased capability is probably the most difficult you've ever had to face.

Reflect

It takes a while, but reflecting on your post-stroke situation is essential. What happened to me? What are the implications? What is the reality I'm now facing? You, first of all, need to grasp your situation before you can move on. Your caregiver, doctor, and neurologist can play key roles in putting your picture together. But you need to ask questions. They don't know where your 'understanding gaps' are.

It's a slow process. You can only integrate your understanding over time. Meanwhile, your brain is busy trying to figure out how to rewire itself. It's exhausting.

- *So far, what's your understanding of what happened?*

- *What's missing? What are the gaps in your understanding?*

Piecing together one part of the puzzle usually leads to a whole set of new questions. And you may have to hear the explanations more than once. Your short-term memory is not likely what it once was.

Most importantly, do not accept anybody's statement about what your limits are. They're just making their best guesses. They don't really know. Neither do you. I have met so many stroke survivors who were told such things as, "You'll never walk again" and so on. **And so many of those limiting statements were proven wrong.**

Have you been told any limiting statements?

- *If so, what were those limiting statements?*
- *Which ones do you accept?*
- *Which ones do you reject and want to work on?*
- *What personal strengths did you discover as you wrestled with all these issues?*

You need to draw deep. You need to call upon your greatest strengths to pull you forward- even to make the smallest step. At first you probably wanted to get back to the person you once were. Then you realized you might not get that far, so you began to adjust your expectations.

- *What have you done to help you cope?*
- *Right now, how enthusiastic are you about increasing your capability?*

- ***What energizes you?***

You've had a chance to reflect on your situation. This step should have clarified the issues you're facing. Moreover, you should have identified the strengths you can apply to carry you through the rest of the RAISE exercise. If so, you're ready to take the next step: Analyze.

Reflect: The Caregiver's Role

The caregiver helps the survivor to reflect on what really happened and to document those reflections. Questioning stimulates the survivor to access these sometimes sensitive and painful memories. The caregiver can also help the survivor fill in a few gaps in understanding and recall. Documenting the reflections helps to 'anchor' them so they can be more easily accessed in the following RAISE steps.

Step 2: Analyze (RAISE)

"The Brain: an apparatus with which we think we think"

(Ambrose Bierce)

Guiding Question:

If this is how the brain works and learns, what am I going to do with mine?

You still have a brain. Well, maybe not all of it- but enough. Enough of a brain to make better use of it than you ever thought.

- *How do you think you can make better use of your brain?*

Let *me* explain. We all know the brain is the most complex organ in the body and is still the least understood. However, breakthroughs in brain imaging have led to extraordinary advances in brain research and therapy in recent years.

How the Brain Works and Learns

It's important for stroke survivors to understand a little about this new knowledge of how the brain works and learns. Why? So we can better learn how to increase our capability as stroke survivors.

- **What do you know about the brain? How does it work and learn?**

Some of us will have great difficulty improving how our brain and body work. At the same time, no medical specialist, researcher or therapist can tell us we've reached the limit of our capability. Let me provide the smallest of examples.

A year and a half after my stroke, I was standing in front of the bathroom mirror, preparing to shave. Normally I would shake the shaving cream with my left hand and arm before wielding the razor with my right hand. However, stroke had impaired my left side. I had trouble 'getting' the right movement, which was to shake the can directly up and down to create the right amount of foam. My hand and arm tended to go around in an oval, so I'd hold onto my left hand with my right to stabilize it. I would even tell my left hand and arm that they were doing a good job.

Then one day as I was getting ready to shave, I noticed my left hand moving deftly up and down-shaking my shaving cream. I couldn't believe it. 'Shake it up, baby!'

Remember, this was a year and a half after my stroke. It was a small thing, but oh so important to me.

- **What special event do you recall that overcame a deficit?**

- ***How did it make you feel?***

So don't ever think there's a limit to what you can do. And recent brain research tells us that there's reason to hope. The brain *can* change, and so can we change our ability!

- ***Do you think you can increase a specific ability? Why?***

Let's walk through a few brain basics so you can better understand how the brain works and learns, what actually happened to you, and what you might do to 'rewire' your brain to 'rewire' your life.

Brain Basics

Before we get underway you need to keep in mind two things: everybody's brain is different; everybody's stroke is different. What really happened to you and what you might do about it are largely unknown. However, you probably have a better idea than anybody else about your situation. You are your own best doctor.

Understanding the brain (and mind) is still in its early stages of research and knowledge. But we have to deal with what we've got. Here we go!

Your brain is loaded with about 100 billion brain cells. They're called neurons. And, on average, each of these cells connects to about 10,000 other neurons in a vast complex called a neural network.

> This three-pound organ is the seat of intelligence, interpreter of the senses, initiator of body movement, and controller of behavior.
>
> ('Brain Basics: Know Your Brain, Introduction,' NINDS website)

The odd thing about the brain is that (as far as we know) there really is no 'content' as such. It's essentially chemistry and configuration- or neurotransmitters and networks.

For example, we really don't yet know how a word or an idea is formed. But through brain imaging devices we're beginning to identify particular networks of neurons which 'light up' in response to the eyes seeing a specific image.

Let's think about parallels.

- *How is the brain similar to something else you're familiar with?*
- *How is the brain different or opposite from anything else you're familiar with?*

The 'Polysensory' Brain

Bach-y-Rita was working with a team of German researchers in the 1960s. "They were studying how vision worked by measuring with electrodes electrical discharge from the visual processing area of a cat's brain." (Doidge, *The Brain That Changes Itself*, p. 17)

When they showed an image to a cat, the electrode showed the cat responding to that image in the visual processing part of the brain. However, when the cat's paw was accidentally touched, "the visual area was also fired, indicating that it was processing touch as well." (Doidge, p. 17) Moreover, when the cat heard sounds, once again the visual processing area reacted.

Bach-y-Rita reflected on the traditional idea of the brain being hardwired- each of its components dedicated to one specialized function. Based upon the research team's experience with the cat, 'localization' didn't seem to make sense.

It was then that Bach-y-Rita "began to conceive of much of the brain as 'polysensory'-that its sensory areas were able to process signals from more than one sense." (Doidge, p. 17) Much more of a 'shared responsibility' than we thought. Breakthrough!

- *If one part of your brain can possibly step in to help a part lost to stroke, what does that mean to you?*

The Brain Over Time

The ability of your brain to change (neuroplasticity) provides the foundation of hope. Recent brain research indicates we are capable of reconfiguring our brain *no matter what our age.*

In the first few years of life, the brain expands.

As the child grows in knowledge and skills, a vast network of neurons (brain cells), axons (senders of information), and dendrites (receivers of information) reach out to other neurons to increase the density and complexity of the child's neural network.

- *As far as you can recall, what was the earliest learning (neural network building) breakthrough for you?*

However, as the child approaches puberty, things start to change. The brain begins to pare down neurons as the adolescent develops keener interest in a few things (the opposite sex, for example), and loses interest in other things (e.g., reciting in front of the class).

The brain responds accordingly. The neural network develops more 'connections' in opposite sex information and knowledge, and loses connections in the ability to recite. So those 'recitation' neurons actually start to weaken and wither. The other ones start to grow.

- *As you went through puberty, how did your interests change?*

- *What childhood 'learnings' (skills and knowledge) did you forget or leave behind?*

- *How did they change again as you became an adult?*

Piaget (a Swiss philosopher) identified four stages of cognitive development in which the brain experiences rapid growth in your younger years. The last one which starts in puberty and stretches into the early twenties he calls the formal operational period. It's characterized by the ability to think abstractly and reason logically.

As a young adult, not only does your reasoning ability grow, but your more specialized neural networks become stronger as you develop specific competencies and skills. However, you also lose some potential to quickly develop other capabilities. That's the trade-off.

- *What trade-offs have you and your brain made?*

The Brain and Learning

As your interests changed, your brain, over time, reconfigures its connections. Your brain becomes increasingly specialized through more focused learning.

- However, the brain still retains its neuroplasticity throughout life
- Owing to its neuroplasticity, the brain builds a denser network of neurons in the parts responsible for specific functions as it learns and responds to life's experiences
- Unlearning precedes new learning first by weakening certain neurons and reconfiguring

a 'new learning' set of neurons- this is somewhat difficult and takes time

• Learning is then anchored by memory

Do you think your brain is flexible enough {neuroplastic) to learn how to improve your capability? Why do you think that?

The important message here is that, based upon recent research, there is significant hope for stroke survivors to improve their capability. Even though, through a stroke, you lost a number of brain cells, certain other parts of your brain might take over some of the 'responsibility' of the lost parts.

'Taking Over'

What is the research showing? The brain is not as hardwired as previously thought. Yes, specific components and areas of the brain do perform specific functions.

For example, the cerebellum (the 'little brain' at the back) takes care of balance and coordination- among other things. If a stroke kills off brain cells (neurons) in that part of our brain, then it's going to be difficult to recover that ability. However, some of that function might be taken over by other parts of our brain- but maybe not as well because they're also busy doing their normal brain stuff.

What's a parallel? Think of a time when a workmate

stepped in to help you get something done (you might have been a little sick). So he was able to take on your workload, but struggled with it. Why? Because he also had his own responsibilities. At the same time, he more or less did get your job done.

- **What is a similar example in your own life?**

'Use It to Improve It'

So in a case of stroke, at least part of your lost capability might be assumed by a part of your brain that performs a similar or related function.

The fear of many stroke survivors is that capability lost can never be regained. So there is a tendency to rely on the obvious and strong capability that remains (e.g., using your strong hand to pick up things- not your weak hand).

Unfortunately, this tendency turns into a vicious cycle. The less you use the weak side, the weaker it becomes. Constant repetition (practice) is needed to improve a particular brain function to overcome a 'deficit.'

There's no guarantee that a stroke survivor can partially or totally overcome a specific handicap, but what do you have to lose? It's worth a try.

- **In your own life, what's an example of 'using it to improve it?'**

For us stroke survivors, the 'using it to improve it' brain principle poses both a hurdle and a hope. If we actively practice or develop a skill such as buttoning a shirt, we will likely maintain or slightly enhance our present capability.

If we let somebody else button our shirt, particularly that last sleeve button on our strong side (requiring our weak side hand to do it), relearning that capability will be more difficult in the future.

- ***What skill or task did you pass to somebody else that you could have done- but was 'easier' if somebody else did it for you?***

Why? Because those button-upping neurons (brain cells) are degenerating ("learned non-use", Taub) and being replaced by neurons busy with something else you *are* doing regularly.

So to rebuild that button-upping capability later will mean 'borrowing' nearby neurons to help out or hoping other neurons will move to the new task. All that takes time and dedicated practice. That's why therapists get you up and goin' right after your stroke- to prevent 'learned non-use.'

Stroke and the Brain

Stroke is caused by either a) blockage of a blood vessel that prevents oxygen and nutrients from reaching the brain or b) rupturing of a blood vessel in the brain that leads to bleeding, damage and pressure on the brain. In either case, it's viewed as a 'brain attack.'

> Since the brain relies on the glucose and oxygen carried by blood cells for energy, brain cells will begin to die after about four minutes without these nutrients.
>
> (Burkman, *The Stroke Recovery Book*, p. 4)

Ischemic strokes, the ones that prevent blood from reaching the brain, come from two sources:

a. thrombosis- the leading cause of stroke, clogs blood vessels with cholesterol or clotted blood (like a drainpipe that becomes thinner and thinner because of lime and other minerals that cling to the insides of the pipe); and
b. embolism- the second leading cause of stroke, comes from a clot breaking off from a blood vessel somewhere in the body that enters the circulatory system in the brain until it reaches an artery it can't pass through.

Hemorrhagic strokes, caused by a bursting blood vessel in the brain, are the most deadly. However, if the patient survives beyond thirty days, there is a good chance of full recovery. They are most often caused by high blood pressure.

About 86% of strokes are ischemic, and 13% hemorrhagic.

- ***What kind of stroke did you have? What was its impact?***

Sometimes after a stroke some dead brain cells are replaced by live and active ones. Such brain capability to change, learn, and rewire itself is called neuroplasticity. This brain malleability has only recently been confirmed by breakthrough brain imaging technology.

These brain imaging devices- EEGs, fMRIs, CT scans, etc.- have stimulated significant brain research. For the first time, researchers can 'see' inside the brain, not just make best guesses. What a difference!

- *Are you excited about the possibilities? Why? (I am.)*

These new brain imaging systems and subsequent research have stimulated the exciting idea of the brain's ability to 'remake' itself. Stroke survivors can now consider how to increase their capability- no matter when they had their stroke.

For some it might mean slightly increasing the dexterity of their fingers; for others it could be taking a little more control of their tongue. For us stroke survivors, any small improvement is deeply felt and valued.

- *What small improvements would make a difference to you?*

Of course, outstanding brain research and breakthrough imaging technology aren't enough. The stroke survivor herself has to draw upon certain strong character traits to guide her through this difficult exercise of rewiring her brain.

Rebuilding Your Brain

However, there is hope. When you start rebuilding your former capability in something, your neurons quickly get to work. In fact, if you use them, your neurons could strengthen in a number of ways:

a. they will thicken;
b. different neuronal rearrangements will take place; and
c. they'll develop greater capability to generate electrical impulses (called 'active potentials') to bridge synapses to other nearby neurons.

Whew! That's a lot of brain work. And *your* brain can still do it. Remember- a hundred billion neurons and trillions of axons can't all be wrong. You didn't lose all of them. So get the remainder back on the job.

- ***Start thinking about areas of lost capability you might partially regain if you worked on them (get other parts of your brain to 'take over'). What are they?***

Stroke affects all of us differently. Different parts of our brain are lost permanently. Some of us lose more than others. Our ability to recover, to some degree, depends on what brain components we lost. Certain components can be more easily 'replaced' by other components. Others are harder to replace. More research needs to be done to clarify the more 'replaceable' parts of the brain.

Replacement

'Replaceable' in this context means that one part of the brain can step in to do some of the work originally done by another part. As mentioned earlier, it rarely does as well. That's because that part is still working on its original function- as well as taking on another function.

In one extreme example, a girl lost one whole hemisphere (her left), but stayed alive. Moreover, her right hemisphere started taking on some of the lost functions of the left hemisphere such as language capability. However, only part of that capability was retained.

So what does all of this mean for stroke survivors?

1. Part of our lost capability can be undertaken by another part of the brain.
2. Some of that lost capability can be regained by 'training' other parts of the brain.
3. We can strengthen brain 'components' just by using them a lot.

In other words, there is much we can do to support our brain's natural ability to 'repair' itself- and perhaps go beyond just repair.

New connections take time to form and strengthen. They gradually learn what is most useful and adapt. Many stroke victims lose language abilities, but neighboring circuits or neurons in the non-damaged hemisphere try to take over and compensate for the lost function.

(Ratey, *A User's Guide to the Brain*, p. 38, 39)

Recovery

The likelihood of recovery from a stroke is largely determined by the extent of damage and location of the stroke.

Therefore, the injury will affect the body functions governed by a particular region. For example, a marble-sized area of damage in the upper cortical levels of the brain may cause weakness in the hand. Yet the same sized damage in the brain stem may result in worse symptoms such as paralysis of an arm or leg because so many more nerves funnel into this area. (Burkman, pp. 71, 72)

However, we're alive, and therefore blessed. We just need to find out how we might improve our capability, even a little, to lead more satisfying and fruitful lives. You *will* need to stretch yourself, and it will take more than a little work.

- ***Think of instances in your past that really challenged you and required your brain to 'stretch' itself. What were they?***

  Activities that challenge your brain actually expand the numbers and strength of neural connections devoted to that skill.

  (Ratey, p. 37)

Now you've had a chance to think about your stroke capability situation, it's time to specifically identify what you want to rebuild.

Analyze: The Caregiver's Role

Obviously the caregiver can't expect to be 'a brain' about the brain. However, the caregiver can provide specific examples of the survivor's brain 'neuroplasticity'- for example, how much the survivor has improved since the day of the stroke.

Any improvement at all illustrates her brain's ability to carve out new neural pathways to compensate for lost capability. Her brain has truly learned. Surely it can learn a little more. The caregiver is now starting to coach the survivor to analyze potential capabilities to work on.

The **Analyze** sub-section, points out to stroke survivors that there is now a scientific or, more properly, a neuroscientific basis for hope. The brain, even after traumatic damage and long term inattention, could still repair itself (with a little help from its owner).

The caregiver's role, then, is to build on that basis for hope so the survivor is motivated and better prepared for the hard work ahead.

Step 3: Identify (RAISE)

"Strength does not come from physical capacity. It comes from an indomitable will."
(Mohandas Ghandi)

Guiding Question:

How can you use your strengths to develop your capability?

In this section, we want you to think about the stories of the strong stroke survivors, their characteristics, and how closely you identify with their strengths. After all, it is these strengths and others that will help you develop your competencies. We'll then ask you to identify what you want to develop in both your plan and practice.

- *What strong stroke survivor strengths have you identified in their stories so far?*

- *Which of these strengths do you identify with? In other words, which of their strengths do you possess? How strong are they in you? Think of things you've done that exhibit those strengths.*

- *What other strengths are carrying you forward?*

Personal Strength

Personal strength seems to come from a number of sources: what you were born with (heredity), obstacles you have overcome, support from family and friends, focus on a specific vision or goal, and spiritual inspiration and belief.

Heredity

Well, you can't do much about this one. Your ancestors did it. That's why it's helpful to dig out the stories of your parents, grandparents, great grandparents, and so on. All had to deal with adversity one way or another- coming to America, pioneering, starting a farm or business, or simply surviving.

- *What relative's story stands out in your mind that showed real strength of character? What was the story? How did it demonstrate strength?*

When I moved to New Jersey, it seemed like a foreign land- dominated by fast-moving traffic on turnpikes whose towns and villages were identified by freeway exit numbers. Initially I came on my own to see how we might settle in our new home. 'Joisey' held such promise and opportunity for my family.

I remember driving down one freeway close to the Hudson River and Manhattan's skyline. I felt like a real pioneer zipping along in the traffic. For some reason one of my grandfathers came to mind. After arriving from England, he worked his way up to become a sea captain and then a pilot, guiding ships into a major harbor on the West Coast.

I could 'see' him, a short, bow-legged captain with his hands clasped behind his back, captain's hat on, riding the sea waves as he surveyed the coastline. On a New Jersey turnpike, you ask? Yes. That vision of him and his 'indomitable will' kept me going as we figured out how to settle in our new land.

Eventually he had a stroke. To look at him, I could never tell. And he never told.

Think about the incredible strength shown by one of your ancestors. *You* have that strength. Use it.

Obstacles

At first, as a stroke survivor, the road ahead seems nothing but terrifying obstacles. You confronted your first obstacle in simply surviving (I was just kidding- I didn't really mean 'simply'). As you learn to overcome each obstacle (for some, it's picking up a fork to eat with) the other ones seem less daunting.

Most of us are faced with a unique set of disabilities. Just figuring out which ones to work on first presents an obstacle. As you move forward to deal with each of them, your inner fiber strengthens.

- ***What's the biggest obstacle you're presently confronting? How do you plan to deal with it or overcome it? What strength will you need?***

Support

It's difficult to go it alone. Even when you have full support of family and friends, sometimes you feel very isolated—that your struggle is strictly a personal struggle. But when you reflect on it, you know those who care about you want to see you through.

This awareness, that others really do care about you, helps to build your personal strength.

- ***How have the care, support, and love you've received made a difference in your recovery?***

Vision or Goal

Some of us kind of muddle through our recovery. However, those who make the most constructive and significant gains are usually people guided by some personal recovery vision or goal. By vision, I mean the survivors who can actually 'see' themselves at the end of their recovery period. They see a whole, or at least a more able, person. Think of Janice.

Others are driven by a specific recovery goal they set for themselves. Think of Tony.

- *Describe the specific recovery vision or goal you set for yourself.*

Spiritual Inspiration and Belief

Many stroke survivors see this source of strength as the most important one in their lives. In some cases, their personal strength is grounded in their religion. For others, it is a general belief that their life is guided by a Supreme Being or spiritual force.

In my own case, I asked myself a hard-to-answer question in my early recovery: Why was I spared? Evidently about 80% of those who had a similar stroke to mine died. Again, why was I spared? I could think of no other answer to that question than the following: I was spared to prevent stroke and help other stroke survivors. This question and answer have guided my life ever since I had a stroke.

- *What kind of spiritual guidance has kept you going?*

Obviously the more sources of personal strength you can draw from, the better opportunity you have to accept or overcome your disabilities.

Identify Your Focus for Improvement

Now it's time to decide what specific capability you want to improve. Maybe you already have a clear idea, and you just want to get on with it. If so, then just skip the rest of this section. However, I caution you. Even if you've already made your final decision, at least consider the 'Focus Guidelines' before you make your final final decision.

You've already assessed your strengths as a stroke survivor. What you haven't assessed is which capability you want to work on. Before you decide, consider the following issues.

Focus Guidelines

Each of us likely has more than one disability or one disability that affects a lot of things in our lives. This is when you need to be clear and specific. For example, I have a problem with my balance. I have other problems as well, but let's examine this one first. My balance disability affects the following things:

- Ability to walk in a straight line
- Ability to carry a glass or cup filled with some liquid (usually coffee or wine) or carry a plate of food with my weak side arm and hand
- Ability to walk up and down stairs
- Ability to walk on uneven ground or steep slopes
- Ability to look up (without getting dizzy)

And so on...

So is my disability 'balance' or one of the things listed above? For the purposes of this exercise, we need to consider something specific like 'ability to carry a plate of food.'

To get clearer, let's call a 'big' disability a disability. Let's call an everyday behavior affected by your big disability a 'competency.' So in the example above, the disability is 'balance,' and one of its corresponding competencies is 'carrying a plate of food.'

Here we go. Find a piece of paper somewhere and make a few notes. Identify your 'big' disabilities on the left side and your corresponding 'missing' competencies on the right side. If you can't write this down, then find somebody who *can* write it down and document it for you:

'Big' Disabilities   'Missing' Competencies

Now you need to make a choice- preferably with your caregiver. Here are a couple of things to consider:

- An identifiable pattern of activity in your life
- The things that really matter to you

Pattern of Activity

Are there activities you engage in on a daily or weekly basis? For example, I write on the computer a number of hours at a time- and virtually every day. Yours may be driving, shopping, feeding the dogs, adjusting the tilt of your bed, etc.

- ***What are your regular activities?***

Working on improving a competence that affects your everyday life could be a worthwhile choice. What would be even better is choosing a competence that you use in more than one kind of activity. Walking in a straight line is such an example (if you're able to walk at all).

You need to walk around your house or apartment to get things done; you need to walk when you're shopping; you need to walk into meeting rooms; and some of you 'walk' your dogs. Those are the activities, but you want to improve a specific competence-walking in a straight line- that will affect all those activities. Moreover, it will keep you from bumping into people and things.

What Really Matters to Me

Think ahead. Let's say you actually could improve in that specific competence you've selected. What difference would it make to you- personally? How would you feel?

If you're unsure about your ability to develop a competence important to you, then choose something else you think you actually can develop.

So, in summary, consider your patterns of activity and what really matters to you before you select the competence.

I have a friend who is also a stroke survivor. He had kept a daily journal for 25 years. Then he had a stroke and could no longer keep up his journal. He basically couldn't write at all.

Although writing in itself was important to him, keeping a journal was **really** important to him. He was motivated to learn how to write again so he could maintain his journal.

- *So, with your caregiver, review your major disabilities and select a corresponding key competence. Consider your patterns of activity and what's really important to you.*

- *Decide what specific 'thing' you want to improve. This 'thing' will constitute the Purpose of your Capability Improvement Plan. What is it?*

So is this the capability you want to work on? Do you draw on it regularly? Is it one that 'crosses' a few of your activities? Is it one you can likely improve (even a little)? Is it one you want to practice so you can improve?

If so, read on. You're about to undertake the hardest part of **RAISE- Start**. You will plan to act and take action (practice for improvement). You can do it!

Identify: The Caregiver's Role

Now the caregiver needs to help the survivor more clearly understand herself, what she is capable of, and what she wants to focus on.

The caregiver can help the survivor draw from

strengths demonstrated by the eleven survivor stories. This is an important first step for the survivor in generating self-confidence for what lies ahead.

The survivor, in this step of **RAISE** also identifies the competency he wants to improve. The caregiver can provide useful feedback on his daily patterns of activity that suggest which general disability and specific competence will make a difference and be important to the survivor.

Step 4: Start (RAISE)

"Success seems to be largely a matter of hanging on after others have let go."

(William Feather)

Guiding Question:

How do you move from motivation to improvement?

(hint: plan and act)

It's easy to let important things slip. After all, there are so many other things in our lives to get done. However, if we want to improve our capability, "it just ain't gonna happen" by itself. We need to be motivated.

Motivation, first of all, is based on hope and confidence: we *hope* to improve and feel *confident* we can do something about it. Without hope, we'll likely do nothing or nothing much. So, where does the hope come from? Well, it's either from your life experience or from information that gives hope.

- *Think of an incident in your past in which hope helped. How did it help?*

Confidence is generated by your previous experience and results. However, it's also bolstered by how you feel about yourself and the support you receive from others.

- ***Think of the same or another incident in which confidence helped. How did it help?***

If you've ever viewed the film, **Rudy**, you'll see and feel how hope and confidence fused together are a powerful force- overcoming one challenge and obstacle after another. **Rudy** is also a true story.

Strong stroke survivors embody hope and confidence. Moreover, they consistently demonstrate, as you might recall, five characteristics:

Realistic: faces up to the changes in one's medical condition and next steps to take

Optimistic and motivated: views the future in a positive light and eager to improve

Purposeful and determined: clear about why one has survived and consistently carries out that purpose

Focused and disciplined: clear about priorities and adhering to a regular schedule to progress

Resilient: recovers from setbacks (mentally, emotionally, or physically)

Most of these strong survivors have suffered setbacks and experienced 'down' times but those never last that long. And it's usually taken a while for them to 'get there,' to become strong stroke survivors. You'll see as you move forward with this program, how it's structured around the characteristics of these strong stroke survivors.

There is simply no point in moving forward with a capability improvement plan if you're not deeply motivated to improve your competence. Remember, you're focusing on the specific competence you identified in the previous section. How motivated are you to improve it?

Motivation is the key to successful capability improvement. Are you really ready? Your caregiver can probably provide a better answer to that question than you can, and may have to make the final judgment simply because she's a little more objective.

You might even want one of your medical professionals to complete the earlier Preliminary Assessment. Then you would have three different viewpoints on whether you're ready or not.

At this point, we'll assume you've identified what you want to work on and verified that you're properly motivated. Now comes the real test: planning and practice. This section is the most important part of the whole handbook.

> ... repetition of exercises cannot be overemphasized... This means practice is important. Caregivers can help patients with exercises outside therapy sessions, *increasing their potential for progress.* (my italics)
>
> (Burkman, pp. 39, 40)

The following capability improvement format is partially based on Edward Taub's 'massed practice' training principles:

> Skill relates to everyday life
> Done in increments
> Done in a short time period
> (Doidge, pp. 155, 156)

NOTE

To date, **RAISE** participants who practiced its concentrated, exercises and who completed the program have averaged a 40+% improvement in some specific capability. If they did it, so can you!

Personal Capability Improvement Plan (3 Weeks)

Write your plan down so you can refer back to it:

- to clarify what you set out to do
- how you were going to do it
- and what capability level you started at

With your caregiver (if you have one), you should do the following:

1. Review the *Preliminary Assessment (already completed)*

2. Develop your *Capability Improvement Plan (below):*

   a. <u>Purpose</u> (why I'm participating in this Plan and Exercise)

   b. <u>Goal(s)</u> (my overall intended outcome)

   c. <u>Measurement(s) Current and Desired</u> (specific outcomes now and in three weeks)

   d. <u>Benefits</u> (what my accomplishments will mean to me)

   e. <u>First Week Exercises</u> (two sets of three rounds each morning and evening- except weekends which will be once a day)- Exercises should relate to Measurements and Goals

   f. <u>Daily Plan</u>

3. Accept feedback and support from your caregiver.

- ***Refer to the Appendix (Personal Capability Improvement Plans) to see how to fill out your planning form. Two examples are provided.***

When you complete the plan, make a contract with yourself (and your caregiver) to carry out the plan to the best of your ability. Write it down or get somebody to write it for you. Sign it, date it, and keep it. Pull it out every week at 'Check-in' to remind yourself about what you're trying to accomplish.

In most cases, you should plan to do two sets of exercises or practices- one in the morning and one in the late afternoon or early evening. Each set of exercises should last no more than 30-45 minutes.

A 'set' will be comprised of three rounds with a short break between each round to regain your energy and focus for the next round. Take your time. Don't proceed until you're ready.

In the exercise format, both morning and evening practice start with meditation and visualization. These key steps relax you, set the tone for your practice and help you 'see' yourself performing successfully. In an experiment Yue and Cole "showed that imagining one is using one's muscles actually strengthens them." (Doidge, p. 204).

At the end of the set, congratulate yourself for doing

the exercise, focusing on your goal, and working hard on improvement. Close your eyes to see yourself 'performing at 'goal' level. Then reward yourself.

Follow exactly the same process in the evening, except conclude by reflecting on what you need to do the next day to increase your capability.

At certain times you will be fatigued, cranky, or just not motivated to do your exercises. Do them anyway. The benefits are tremendous. Keep reminding yourself.

> Changing the brain's firing patterns through repeated thought and action ...is responsible for the initiation of self-choice, freedom, will, and discipline.
>
> (Ratey, p. 36)

In Summary

You probably noted the suggested Daily Plan is for only the first week. At the end of that week, you need to sit down with your caregiver to review the week's results and develop a plan for the second week. At the end of the second week you review how you did and then plan for the third and final week.

You and the caregiver might decide to carry on with the same exercises and measurements through the entire three weeks. Or, you might want to make adjustments. However, be careful about making adjustments. If the initial goals are

worthy goals, you should probably stay with them
and not back off.

Exercises and measurements are another matter.
In the first week you were basically experimenting,
trying things out. Now you know better. You may
choose another set of exercises and/or measurements
for a variety of reasons:

- You want to RAISE the level or standard each
  week
- You want a varied set of exercises (less
  boring)
- One or more of the exercises didn't 'work'
- One or more of the measurements didn't
  'work'
- Timing was off- too many sets of exercises, too
  much time consumed, too little energy, etc.

You need to find a balance between challenge and
maintenance, between risk and security. Keep
working at it. You and your caregiver are building
your unique pathway through the woods.

After you've actually planned and worked on your
RAISE program, ask yourself: How did I do? Did I
actually improve my capability? If so, how much?
And so on... These are the next steps.

Start: The Caregiver's Role

The caregiver plays *the* key role in **Start**. This is
when the caregiver truly becomes 'coach.'

Here are the tasks the caregiver needs to undertake:

- Help the survivor complete the **Preliminary Assessment.**
- Review the results together—determine whether or not the survivor is motivated enough to complete the three week program.
- If so, help the survivor complete the **Personal Capability Improvement Plan (3 weeks)**.

  o *Purpose* is more general (improve balance) than specific *Goals* (able to walk in a straight line, able to carry a glass of water without spilling it, able to step over cords on the floor without falling).

  o *Measurements* refers to the specific ways you'll determine a capability—before the practice sessions (*Current Capability)* and after them (*Desired Capability*). Select, with the survivor, at least two, but no more than four measurements. The measurements could be 'hard' or 'soft'—preferably both. 'Hard' refers to quantitative measures such as speed or distance. 'Soft' measures could include such things as quality or success. The measures could be made by either caregiver or survivor herself. Exactly the same measures will be used before and after, although we would expect different results! Sometimes a little creativity is required here. In certain cases, rough estimates might be the only solution.

o ***Current Capability*** is determined by actually applying the measurements (How long did he take? How far did she go?).

o ***Future Capability*** is determined by the specific, challenging, but reasonable goals of the survivor- how much she wants to improve in three weeks' time. The same measurements used to measure current capability will be used to measure future capability.

o ***First Week Exercises*** flow from everything else, particularly from the measurements used. The survivor will mentally 'warm up' (by briefly meditating and visualizing) for about 10 minutes. No more than two to four exercises should be undertaken in each session.

Keep in mind, however, that three rounds of these exercises will be practiced in both morning and late afternoon/early evening (only one session on Saturdays and Sundays).

A brief 'breather' is taken between each round. These three rounds of exercises should take no longer than 30 to 45 minutes. The caregiver helps the survivor walk through these steps until he can do them on his own (if that is possible).

o **Review Morning's Performance and Weekly Goal** with the survivor. Survivor takes the lead and coach prompts. You, as coach, also need to provide honest feedback and encouragement. Any progress towards the goal needs to be recognized and rewarded.

This also is the time to make any suggestions on how performance could be improved. Remind the survivor of the weekly goal and progress made toward it. Sometimes progress in attitude should be noted.

o **Congratulations** are in order just because the survivor had the discipline to try the exercises. However, don't overdo it. The focus is on improved performance and attaining that personal goal. Reinforce those objectives.

o **Visioning** is done by the survivor alone. Just remind her to do it. Visioning focuses, eyes closed, on the survivor seeing herself performing at the level of her personal goal.

Sometimes this will work, other times not. That's all right. At least visioning gives the survivor the chance to reflect on her performance improvement.

o **Rewarding** is important. It could be something as simple as a fresh cup of coffee or going outside to look at the birds in the bird feeder- whatever works for the survivor at that moment. Just make sure he does it, and help him do it. He deserves it.

o *Late Afternoon/Evening Exercises* parallel those of the morning, except that upon completion, the survivor should reflect for a few minutes on what she wants to achieve the next day.

Encourage her to do that reflection. It links today with tomorrow- a continuous set of exercises and practicing that point toward a personal goal.

*Review the survivor's 'In Summary' (p.116). It will guide you, as a caregiver, on how to proceed in the second and third weeks of the program.

The caregiver should not 'overdo' his role as he works with the survivor over this three week period. The survivor should be encouraged to do as much as he can on his own. This approach obviously builds more independence. The minimal time spent with the survivor would look like the following:

• Helping the survivor develop her Personal Capability Improvement Plan. Suggestions of potential exercises or measurements are particularly helpful. This planning session will probably take about two hours.

• Meeting with the survivor at the end of

each week to do a check-in. This meeting should allow the survivor to share both accomplishments and difficulties with her caregiver. The caregiver might also suggest any needed changes in exercises, measurements or time allotted to the sessions. The check-in will take about an hour.

• Conducting a final assessment session. This session will be explained more fully in the last step, Evaluate. The final assessment may take as long as two hours.

Check-in

Check-in with the survivor needs to be handled with great sensitivity. The survivor has expended a lot of energy in just surviving. Trying to regain part or the whole of a specific competency through concentrated practice and repetition takes a high level of commitment and discipline. Your survivor needs to be commended for that alone.

Begin the feedback session (at the end of the first and second weeks after start-up) with a strong compliment to the survivor for persevering to this point, and reaffirm her desire to achieve her goal.

Then ask her how she thinks she has done. Keep the discussion open-ended. Anything could 'pop up' that deserves further exploration. Certain issues, however, need to be discussed:

a. whether or not the specific exercises should be maintained or changed
b. whether or not the measurements need to be changed
c. how you as caregiver could be more helpful

Goals are a different thing. Try to keep the goals from being changed unless there is a very good reason. In fact, reaffirm the goals in order to remind the survivor that's what she's aiming for.

Basically let the survivor lead the discussion. Your role is to listen carefully, support the survivor's efforts, and make appropriate suggestions when asked.

In Summary

Over the period of three weeks the caregiver commits to approximately five hours of coaching time. The survivor values these few hours together.

However, at times the survivor will find it difficult to do the exercises owing to fatigue, involvement with other activities, or a general feeling of lack of progress. At these times, the caregiver needs to find a balance between reinforcement of the survivor's goals and efforts and forgiveness of any lapses.

Step 5: Evaluate (RAISE)

"Lasting accomplishment... is still achieved through a long slow climb and self-discipline."

(Helen Hayes)

Guiding Question:

How did I do?

So you have finished your three week capability program. Whew! Tough stuff.

Step 1

- *How do you feel about what happened? How did you do?*
- *What was the toughest part? Why?*
- *What was the easiest part? Why?*
- *What did you learn?*

Now it's time to measure how you did. Obviously you need to test yourself again so you can compare your results now with those from your earlier test. Then you'll measure your raw improvement score as well as the percentage of improvement. Hey, maybe you didn't improve. So what! We'll discuss that later. Let's do the measurement first.

At this point, I would advise getting a few sheets of paper and a pen to record all you need to record and calculate all you need to calculate about your accomplishments.

Step 2

Go back to the original thing(s) you wanted to improve (in the **Identify** section) and the goals you set for yourself in the **Capability Improvement Plan.**

Write those down (**Original Purpose** and **Goals**).

Step 3

Refer to the **Start Step** to find a list of your measures and previous results (from your first 'test') and make a note of them.

Then measure again. This is the post 'test.' Use exactly the same measures and tests you used the first time. Start by 'envisioning' your post results before you begin the tests.

Ask your caregiver to help out with the tests so that they can be fair and accurate. Don't worry. We trust you. It's just hard to do the tests and measure yourself at the same time.

Time to compare. List the measures, pre-test results,

and post-test results. Subtract the difference and indicate whether it's a gain (+) or a loss (-).

Let's use typing speed as an example. If pre-test results showed a speed of 20 words per minute (wpm) and post-test results were 25 wpm, then obviously there was a 5 wpm gain (+) representing a 25% improvement (5/20).

List **Measures, Pre-Test and Post-Test Scores, Gain/Loss, and Percent Gain/Loss** beside one another. Then put your measurement numbers under each heading and average the ;percent gain or loss.

Step 4

Review these results with your caregiver. You may want to consider the following questions on your own before meeting with your caregiver. Or, perhaps you want to work on them with your caregiver. Your choice.

- *What are the results telling you?*

- *How do you feel about the results?*

- *Ask your caregiver for specific feedback. What things did he/she notice as you worked on your specific competency?*

With your caregiver discuss your strengths that surfaced during this exercise—and also what still needs to be worked on.

- **What surfaced as your strengths during this exercise? What do you still need to work on?**

Now it's time to reward yourself- regardless of your results. You gave it your best shot. You did the best you could. Moreover, you stayed with it even during the most difficult times. So celebrate with your caregiver. You did it together!

In these concentrated last three weeks you've likely shown a little improvement in some area of your capability. Maybe not.

Either way, you need to carry on with your practicing. It doesn't need to be as intense or regular, but it still needs to be done. Practice, practice, practice. It never ends.

- **By the way, what's the next thing you want to work on?**
- **When will you start?**

The Caregiver's Role: Evaluate

The caregiver plays a central role in helping the survivor through this final RAISE step. The survivor will likely find these steps tiresome and boring. Not the end results, however. These results are what the survivor has been striving for over the last three weeks.

So you'll have to be patient with your survivor as you walk her through the steps measuring capability, comparing capability, and working out the percentages.

Coach your survivor through **Evaluate**.

Step 1: Ask your survivor the four preliminary questions and make a note of the responses for later referral.

Step 2: Ask your survivor to recall the original purpose and goals of his/her RAISE program. Remind, if necessary.

Step 3: Conduct the post-test using the same measures as before. Record the measures, pre and post-test results and calculate the gain and percentage gain. If there is more than one measure, calculate the overall (average) percent gain.

Step 4: Review these results with your survivor; use the above stated questions as a guide for your discussion about the results.

REWARD YOURSELVES!

Summary Points

- **Caregivers: Keep helping your survivor increase capability.**
- **Survivors: Keep rewiring your brain. You will rewire your life!**

ENDNOTE

I need your feedback. Tell me whether or not **RAISE** worked for you. Tell me how **RAISE** could be changed to make it work better for you and other stroke survivors. I need you to help me help other stroke survivors. Your feedback on **RAISE** will help all of us take another step forward in our journey of recovery.

Send your feedback on **RAISE** to:

Bob Guns
345 N. Academy St.
Mooresville, NC 28115
Phone: (609) 879-1023
Email: bob.guns@mi-connection.com

I had to get this handbook out as soon as I could after I found out there was more **hope** for all of us than we had ever expected. If there's any chance of improving even a small bit of our capability *now*, it's worth taking that chance. However, it simply might not work for certain people—except that I have no idea who those certain people are.

Until I tried the program myself, I didn't know whether it would work or not for me. I was startled by the results.

I was even more stunned when Charles, a 79-year-old stroke survivor, told me halfway through his RAISE program that he had just written 19 pages in his journal. He hadn't written a thing since his stroke two years ago because of a stiffened arm and hand.

In my own case, I hadn't completely given up hope about further recovery. There just seemed to be too many battles to fight all at once. I accepted that my current level of recovery was about the best I could do. Little did I know.

It's especially difficult to improve when nobody is suggesting you can do any better than you're already doing.

The whole message here is one of HOPE- hope for you, hope for me, hope for countless others. Let's just figure out a way to foster that hope, get survivors believing in themselves once again, and turn that hope into reality.

I believe we should dare to RAISE hope. And then act on that hope.

The RAISE Program

The three week RAISE Capability Improvement program is offered once a month to interested stroke survivors.

Contact is maintained via email and phone during the self-improvement process. A minimum of five direct contacts are made to:

   a. *Conduct a self-assessment and set-up*
   b. *Plan for specific capability improvement*
   c. *Check in at end of first week*
   d. *Check-in at end of second week*
   e. *Conduct final evaluation*

For those strongly affected by aphasia, webcam and instant messaging can be used.

RAISE program participants receive a free copy of both the handbook and workbook.

If the stroke survivor has a caregiver, that person's active participation in the program is encouraged.

For more information or to register, contact:

>   *Bob Guns, Ph.D.*
>   *bob.guns@mi-connection.com*
>   *609-879-1023*

   * *For those who are financially challenged, special arrangements can be made.*

APPENDIX

- **Examples of Personal Capability Improvement Plans**

Personal Capability Improvement Plan:
Bob Guns

Introduction

The preceding sections of the handbook outline how you could develop a Capability Improvement Plan. Here's how I put mine together. It might give you an idea of how to put yours together.

In the following pages I have illustrated only the key elements of my Personal Capability Improvement Plan. However, before you begin **S**tart, complete **all** the preceding steps:

Reflect
Analyze
Identify

These are the **S**tart components I selected to share with you:

- Preliminary Assessment (earlier version)
- Personal Capability Improvement Plan
- Initial Measurement
- Final Measurement

Like most of you, there were a number of disabilities I could have chosen to work on. However, I decided on my computer keyboard skills. After my stroke, I could barely use my left hand on the keyboard. I was determined to use all my fingers, but I was very slow and made a lot of mistakes. Although I gradually improved, somehow I knew I could do better.

My Motivation Assessment

I do a lot of writing on the computer- particularly related to stroke matters. If I were able to improve my speed and reduce my error rate, I could become a lot more efficient and effective. So I chose improving my keyboard skills.

However, I wanted to check on my motivation. If it wasn't strong enough, I'd move on to one of my other disabilities. So I completed the Motivation Assessment (an earlier version of the Preliminary Assessment). You'll see the results below. In reviewing my results, my caregiver and I felt I was properly motivated.

My Personal Capability Improvement Plan

As you can see below the **Motivation Assessment**, I also completed My **Personal Capability Improvement Plan**. The **Plan** really helped me to clarify what I was trying to do and how I was going to do it. I completed it before I met with my caregiver and reviewed it with her.

I realized upon signing the **Plan**, I was fully committing to it and had to carry it out. My caregiver also signed the **Plan**. I gulped.

The Initial Measurement

The criteria for measuring my progress grew out of my goal: to increase my typing speed and make fewer errors in order to improve my productivity. Looking at the keyboard was secondary.

In the old days this was an important skill because secretaries, in particular, needed to be reading a document while typing it. Switching back and forth from keyboard to document would slow them down.

I included this measure (not looking at the keyboard) because I used to be able to 'touch type' and I wanted to regain that skill. However, later on, I realized 'touch typing' wasn't really that important to me. My writing (typing) rarely involved copying documents. We now use copiers or scanners for that. So I dropped that measure.

The key here is to be committed and flexible at the same time. You need to be committed to carrying out the plan but flexible enough to change your measures as you see fit.

Between Initial and Final Measurement

I measured my speed and error rate after every practice, twice a day for three weeks. I didn't include the results of those measures here because I didn't think they would be that meaningful to you.

Your decision to measure yourself every day is up

to you. If you're simply curious, go ahead and do it. However, beware. Your progress will vary from day to day. Some days you will go backwards. Overall, your trend will likely be upwards, as mine was. Measuring once a week should be sufficient.

I also met with my caregiver at the end of each week to review my progress and discuss my measures and measurements.

The Final Measurement

I completed the Final Measurement the day after my three week program had ended. I shared the final measurement results with my caregiver, and we compared them with the initial results. We were more than pleased.

I had set a goal of 25 words per minute and achieved 27.7 wpm. I had also set a goal of 1.5 errors for every two lines. I achieved .33 errors for 6 lines!

In comparing the Initial Measurement with the Final Measurement, I had improved my speed 43% (8.4/19.3) and my error rate 86% (2/2.3). I didn't measure whether or not I looked at the keyboard because I had abandoned that measurement as no longer relevant to my goal.

Additional Comments

In reviewing how you put everything together, you need to construct a direct link between your **Purpose, Goals, Measurements, and Exercises**.

When you convene the summary meeting with your caregiver, you both should feel that what was achieved directly fulfills your **Purpose**.

You and your caregiver might need to use a little imagination in coming up with measures and exercises. And if your measures are a little crude, fuzzy or inexact, don't worry about it. Both of you just need to feel reasonably confident at the program's end that you've made some measurable progress and hopefully achieved your goals.

Motivation Assessment

1. What keeps you going from day to day?

Starting with, 'Thank you God for this day. Thank you, God.' Also, realizing how much meaningful work I have to do that day keeps me going.

2. Do you feel as if you could increase your capability?

Yes, I'm confident I can increase my capability. I just don't know how much. I also realize it will take focus and discipline.

3. Why do you think you could increase it?

I have seen other increases in my capability, even in my keyboard skills.

4. What will motivate you to increase it?

Seeing that I'm committed enough to give it a try and stay with it. After all, it's only three weeks of my life.

5. If you do increase your capability, how will that:

a. help yourself?

It will increase my confidence and productivity.

a. help others?

Much of my work focuses on stroke prevention and support. My keyboard skills will help me be more efficient and productive in getting that work done.

6. What will reinforce and keep you motivated (both during and after the intense practice)?

Knowing that the outcome I'm trying to achieve and sustain will be well worth it.

7. If you don't increase your capability during the intense practice, will you still be motivated to improve?

In some cases it just takes more time. In other cases there can be a sudden breakthrough. Either one is a possibility.

My Three Week Personal Capability Improvement Plan

Purpose: To improve computer keyboard skills

Measurement: To improve each of the following:
- Increase typing speed to 25 words/minute
- Reduce error rate to 1.5 errors/every 2 lines
- Significantly improve 'touch' skills- only occasionally glancing at the keyboard while typing

Benefit: I spend a lot of time at the keyboard engaged in various tasks, particularly writing. If I could improve my keyboard skills, and thereby reduce the time needed to complete my tasks, I would have appreciably more time to focus on other high priority goals and plans. In the end, I would feel more productive and fulfilled.

Plan:

Preliminary

1. Complete my *Motivation Pre-Assessment*
2. Measure my *Current Capability*
3. Review with my caregiver:
    a) Motivation Pre-Assessment
    b) Purpose
    c) Measurements- Present and Goal
    d) Benefits
    e) Plan
4. Accept support from my caregiver.

Daily Plan

<u>Morning</u>

1. Meditate for 10 minutes.
2. For 5 minutes, close my eyes and 'see' myself typing quickly, virtually error-free, without looking at the keyboard.
3. Practice typing the 'quick brown fox' three times:
   - First time focus on speed
   - Second time focus on errors.
   - Third time focus on not looking at keyboard
4. Briefly break between each round to relax and take a few deep breaths.
5. Repeat these rounds for 1.5 hours.
6. When two hours is almost up, review morning's performance and 3 week goal.
7. Congratulate myself for:
     Doing the exercise
     Focusing on my goal
     Working hard on improvement
8. Close my eyes for five minutes and 'see' myself performing at 'goal' level.
9. Reward myself.

<u>Evening</u>

1. Meditate for 10 minutes.
2. For 5 minutes, close my eyes and 'see' myself typing quickly, virtually error-free, without looking at the keyboard.

3. Practice typing the 'quick brown fox' three times:
   a. First time focus on speed.
   b. Second time focus on errors.
   c. Third time focus on not looking at the keyboard.
2. Briefly break between each round to relax and take a few deep breaths.
3. Repeat these rounds for 1.5 hours.
4. When two hours is almost up, review evening's performance and 3 week goal.
5. Congratulate myself for:
   a. Doing the exercise
   b. Focusing on my goal
   c. Working hard on improvement
8. Close my eyes for five minutes and 'see' myself performing at 'goal' level.
9. Reflect on what I need to do tomorrow to increase capability.
10. Reward myself.

Sample Initial Measurement

The quick, brown fox jumped over the lzy dod.
The quick brown fox jumped over the lazy dog.
The

Initial Measurement 1: 19 words in one minute, two mistakes in 2 lines and continuous looking at keyboard

The quidk brown fox jumped over the lazy dog.
The quidk brown fox jumped over the lazy dog.
The qu

Initial Measurement 2: 20 words per minute, two mistakes in two lines, and looking at keyboard almost all the time

The quick hrown fos jumped over the lazy dog.
The quick brown fox jumped over the lazy dog.
The

Initial Measurement 3: 19 words/minute, 3 mistakes in 2 lines, mostly looking at the keyboard

Average: 19.3 wpm, 2.3 errors/passage, almost continuous viewing of keyboard

{The quidk htrot3n goss jumped obvrgtg tgher lay dobg.
Yhjr auifk bntown fox jumprf obrg hjhr lzzy fob./]

HJjr siofl}

Initial Measurement 4 (no looking at keyboard, trying for speed): 20 so-called words, unlimited errors- 20 per line}

Final Measurement

Integrated (Speed and Error Rate)

The quick brown fox jumps over the lazy dog. The quick brown fox jumps over the lazy dog. The quick brown fox jumps oveer the lazy dog. The quick (29) (1) (Overseeing)

I am so impressed with the people I've interviewed for this handbook. They're all so positive and determined to carry on and do better. (24) (0) (Overseeing)

The quick brown fox jumps over the lazy dog. The quick brown fox jumps over the lazy dog. The quick brown fox jumps over the lazy dog. The quick brown (30) (0) (Viewing and overseeing)

Average: 27.7 wpm, .33 errors/passage, basically overseeing keyboard

Overall Improvement: 43% gain in speed (19.3 wpm- 27.7 wpm), 86% reduction in errors (2.3/ passage- .33/passage)

Personal Example 2:
Charles Memrick- Strong Stroke Survivor

Introduction

Charles is 80 years old, and a special person to his family and friends. He had his stroke three years ago, and is still in the early stages of recovery.

He learned how to make ropes out of grocery bags. Charles strung these over his bed and through his main living area to the bathroom. That's how he gets around. I call him Tarzan.

He had kept a daily journal for 25 years until his stroke. Since then Charles hasn't been able to write. His right arm and hand are stiff and virtually paralyzed.

Charles wanted to start writing again so he could record his daily activities and thoughts in his journal. I decided to give him a hand. Well, actually, I wasn't alone. It was a small group that included Charles himself; his daughter, Julie; his son-in-law, Al; and two of his best friends. Charles had a caregiving team. That helps.

So we (Julie and I) tested Charles' motivation for what lay ahead. You'll see the results below. He was ready.

Then we worked on his Plan. His overall purpose? To get back to interacting and writing. For Charles, interacting included writing. His children and grandchildren would be able to read his journal.

That's interacting- at least part of it. His goal? Any kind of improvement in his writing, which at best, was crude scrawling. See below.

Now the difficult part. Figuring out how to test and measure his skills and set goals and appropriate exercises. All of it took a lot of discussion and an ounce or two of creativity. Julie and I were working with him.

Measures, Goals, Tests, and Exercises

We set up tests that would not only help us measure his skills but also form the basis for exercises:

a. feeling in his arm (which had to be warmed up first)
b. assembly of Russian nesting dolls (finger dexterity)
c. penmanship:
 i) copying strokes (basics of penmanship)
 ii) writing (printing) lines—"The quick brown fox jumps over the lazy dog."

	His goals?	**His initial tests?**
a) arm (quality):	4/10	3/10
b) nesting dolls (speed):	60 sec.	70 sec.
c) copying strokes (quality)	5/10	3/10
d) writing lines (speed)	1 min.	1:50 sec.

Speed was important in some tests, quality in others. The quality judgments were made by Charles alone. He also needed something to warm up his arm. I loaned him my random orbital sander. The vibration would help to get his 'arm going.' We also used these tests as his exercises.

Charles decided he could do only one set of exercises a day (with 3 repetitions). He slept the rest of the day.

Then Charles, Julie, and I signed and dated the contract. The contract had a high impact on Charles. He felt committed. Charles kept a copy.

Progress

After the initial meeting with Charles and Julie, his daughter, I arranged two further meetings- a half time review and a final review. Meanwhile, Julie would drop by every two or three days to see how her father was doing.

At 'mid-term review' (about 10 days later) Charles was making significant progress. He also kept accurate records of his exercises, numbering and dating each one.

However, he had started to 'wander' from his exercises and began to do some creative writing (printing). He even doodled in the margins. We wanted him to keep practicing his penmanship exercises, but he complained, claiming that his overall goal was to write again—and that's what he'd started to do- even if it took two hands to do it.

Final Review

A few days before the final review, Charles told me he had written 19 pages in his journal- and with one hand! I had a hard time comprehending what Charles just told me. I also had a hard time believing it, but I was excited for him and told him so.

At the final review, Charles talked about being surprised, motivated, and excited about his progress. "I think I did spectacular." The toughest part was trying to discipline himself. The easiest was just doing the penmanship exercises.

What did Charles learn? "That if you don't continue to keep your body engaged and active, you lose the ability to function."

Charles improved:

- arm quality: **100%**—from 3/10 to 6/10
- nesting dolls speed: **60%**—from 70 sec. to 28 sec.
- penmanship strokes quality: **167%**—from 3/10 to 8/10
- his writing speed: **30%**—from 1:50 to 1:18 sec.

Overall improvement?   **89% in three weeks. Moreover, he was writing every day in his journal which was his long term ambition.** Spectacular results.

Summary

Charles learned that he's capable of discipline if he's motivated. Julie, his caregiver, was impressed that her father did it every day. He didn't need prompting or a reward. It was "something that fed his soul."

Julie felt that her father wanted to improve. He expressed something about himself through the exercise and trusted us (his caregiving team). Charles still wants to work on the quality of his penmanship. However, he doesn't want to speed it up because his thoughts are too slow.

Charles claims he was "jump started- just like an engine." Although he's still not satisfied with his penmanship, he "upped it over and above what he set out to do." He wants to "keep his engine running and synchronize his thoughts and creativity with his hand speed."

Charles said he "wouldn't have done any of this if people didn't care."

Handwriting Examples of Charles' Initial and Final Measurements

Initial Handwriting Measurement

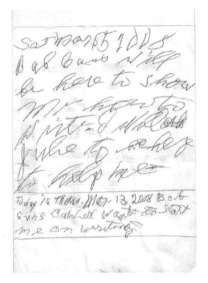

Final Handwriting Measurement

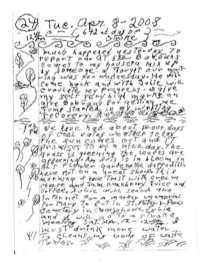

Bibliography

Amen, Daniel G. *Change Your Brain, Change Your Life: The Breakthrough Program for Conquering Anxiety, Depression, Obsessiveness, Anger, and Impulsiveness.* New York: Three Rivers Press, 1998.

Begley, Sharon. *Train Your Mind. Change Your Brain: How A New Science Reveals Our Extraordinary Potential to Transform Ourselves.* New York: Ballantine, 2007.

Burkman, Kip. *The Stroke Recovery Book: A Guide for Patients and Families.* Omaha: Addicus Books, 1998.

Carter, Rita. *Mapping the Mind.* Berkley: University of California Press, 1998.

Dispenza, Joe. *Evolve Your Brain: The Science of Changing Your Mind.* Deerfield Beach, Florida: Health Communications, Inc., 2007.

Doidge, Norman. *The Brain that Changes Itself: Stories of Personal Triumph from the Frontiers of Brain Science.* New York: Viking, 2007.

Gellatly, Angus & Zarate, Oscar. *Introducing Mind &*

Brain: A Graphic Guide to the Science of Your Grey Matter. Cambridge, UK: Icon Books, 2007.

Gibb, Barry J. *The Rough Guide to the Brain: Get to Know Your Grey Matter.* London: Rough Guides Ltd., 2007.

Hinds, David M. *After Stroke.* London: Thorsons, 2000.

Hutton, Cleo. *After a Stroke: 300 Tips for Making Life Easier.* New York: Demos Medical Publishing, 2005.

Johnson, Steven. *Mind Wide Open: Your Brain and the Neuroscience of Everyday Life.* New York: Scribner, 2004.

Kandel, Eric R. *In Search of Memory: The Emergence of a New Science of the Mind.* New York: Norton, 2006.

LeDoux, Joseph. *Synaptic Self: How Our Brains Become Who We Are.* New York: Penguin, 2002.

Medina, John. *Brain Rules: 12 Principles for Surviving and Thriving at Work, Home, and School.* Seattle: Pear Press, 2008.

Ratey, John J. *A User's Guide to the Brain: Perception, Attention, and the Four Theaters of the Brain.* New York: Vintage, 2002.

Robinson, Robin. *Peeling the Onion: Reversing the*

Ravages of Stroke, A Father/Daughter Journey Through a Revolutionary Medical Treatment for Stroke. Key West, Florida: SORA Publishing, 2005.

Siegel, Daniel J. *The Mindful Brain: Reflections and Attunement in the Cultivation of Well-Being.* New York: Norton, 2007.

Siles, Madonna. *Brain, Heal Thyself: A Caregiver's New Approach to Recovery from Stroke, Aneurysm, and Traumatic Brain Injuries.* Charlottesville, VA: Hampton Road Publishing, 2006.

Stroke Associations

- **American Stroke Association**
  - o Are you at risk? Controllable and un-controllable risks. How to recognize a stroke. American Stroke Association National Center
    - 7272 Greenville Ave.
    - Dallas, TX 75231-4596
    - 1-888-4-STROKE
    - www.AmericanStroke.org

- **American Stroke Foundation**
  - o Aims to increase awareness of "Brain Attack" at all levels. A national voluntary health care organization focusing on stroke prevention, treatment, rehabilitation.
    - American Stroke Foundation
      5960 Dearborn, Suite 100
      Mission, KS 66202
      913-649-1776
      Toll-free: 1-866-549-1776
    - www.strokecenter.org

- **National Institute of Neurological Disorders and Stroke**
  The primary NIH organization for research on stroke. Also called Brain Attack Coalition.
  - o NINDS
    Building 31, Room 8A-16

31 Center Drive, MSC2540
Bethesda, MD 20892
301-496-5751
- www.ninds.nih.gov

- **National Stroke Association**
  o Information on stroke, stroke prevention, stroke recovery, and stroke care
  o National Stroke Association
    9707 E. Easter Lane
    Centennial, CO 80112
    1-800-STROKES (1-800-787-6537)
    - www.stroke.org

Stroke Support Websites

H.O.P.E. for Stroke: www.hope4stroke.com

Medline Plus (Stroke):
www.nlm.nih.gov/medlineplus/stroke.html

Stroke Connection Magazine:
www.strokeassociation.org

StrokeNet Message Board: www.strokeboard.net

Strokes Suck: www.strokessuck.com

The Stroke Association: www.stroke.org.uk

The Stroke Network: www.strokenetwork.org

Alternative Stroke Therapies

A few alternative stroke therapies are outlined below. These different therapeutic approaches appear to offer some hope for stroke survivors. However, the author is not recommending any of these approaches. The decision to undertake a particular therapy is a highly individual and personal one. As before, we STRONGLY RECOMMEND you consult with your physician or neurologist before undertaking any of these therapies.

Conventional stroke therapies include physical therapy, occupational therapy, and speech therapy. However, a broader range of stroke therapies is available to survivors, and a few are based on recent neuroscientific research. Only a small sample of these disparate approaches is outlined below, but enough for you to consider alternatives to therapies you've already tried.

Aerobic Exercise

Aerobic exercise appears to be directly linked to brain stimulation and development of long term memory. Evidently aerobic exercise increases levels of BDNF, a neurotransmitter "which encourages neurons to form new synapses and strengthen existing ones." (p. 69, Newsweek, Dec. 10, 2007, "Jogging Your Memory," Anne Underwood) Carl Cotman, director of the Institute for Brain Aging and Dementia at UC Irvine, calls BDNF 'brain fertilizer.'

Another study at Columbia involving aerobic exercise "led to brain scans that seemed to indicate the birth of new neurons in the hippocampus." (p. 69, Newsweek). Through aerobic exercise, Barry Gordon, founder of the memory clinic at Johns Hopkins contends that "with a reasonable amount of effort, you can improve your memory 30 to 40%." (p. 69, Newsweek)

A more specialized form of aerobic exercise is conducted in swimming pools. Benefits for stroke survivors are based on a balance between support and resistance in the water. Training focuses on a range of exercises that improve posture, balance, strength/ endurance, range of motion, weight management, coordination/agility and strengthening of heart and lungs. And for many people, it's simply fun.

Memory Workouts

The brain's 'use it to improve it' principle appears to have been confirmed in a study conducted by Peter Penzes at Northwestern University. The study showed "that brain activity boosts the function of a protein called kalarin-7, whose function had been unclear. Penzes demonstrated that kalarin enlarges and strengthens synapses. By contrast, blocking kalarin causes synapses to shrink." (p. 69, Newsweek)

A brain exercise program developed by Posit Science was tested on 524 adults 65 and over. It involved working an hour a day for eight weeks on a computer-based learning program that demonstrated improvements in a variety of unrelated memory tasks. However, it's unknown how long the benefits of this program will last.

Constraint-Induced Therapy

Constraint-Induced Therapy (CIT) was pioneered by Edward Taub who now heads up a clinic at the University of Alabama in Montgomery. CIT is based on the notion that constraining the use of the survivor's 'good arm' or 'good leg' forces use of the weak arm or leg. Coupled with exercises based on everyday activities and intensive coaching, CIT shows physical capability improvement within a two to three week period regardless of how long ago a stroke occurred.

Biofeedback

Biofeedback visually reinforces moving your arms or hands in the 'right way.' It has proved more helpful in developing fine muscle control than in developing functional use such as using a pen.

> In biofeedback, a wire electrode connected to a metal plate is attached to the skin over an arm or leg muscle. When the survivor moves this muscle, an electrical signal travels from the electrode to an attached monitor, where it produces a particular image. The survivor gets reinforcement every time he or she moves the muscle and creates this image... 'After a stroke, it is common for survivors to move their

arms or legs abnormally, says Dr. Richard L. Harvey, medical director of the Stroke Rehabilitation Center at the Rehabilitation Institute of Chicago. 'Biofeedback can train a survivor to move more naturally.' ("A Rehab Revolution," Stroke Connection Magazine, September/October, 2004)

Functional Tone Management Arm Training

F.T.M. uses an orthotic that enables patients to open and close their hands and handle objects. Concentrated and repetitive practice sessions (up to 250-400 repetitions) with this spring-loaded, mechanical device are used to overcome tightening of the muscles and tendons and learned non-use of the affected hand.

> Kim McKenzie was 21 years post-stroke when she started the program. Before she started, she could not open her hand and fingers. After a week of therapy, she regained hand and finger movement. One year after his stroke, John Gooden recovered movement in one hand and fingers after using the orthotic for 45 minutes three times a week, for three weeks. (From an article, "A Rehab Revolution," Stroke Connection Magazine, September/October, 2004)

The orthotic, developed by two occupational therapists, is now called Saebo-Flex and is FDA approved for outpatient use.

Other Therapies

An extensive range of other therapies could be explored, such as acupuncture and hyperbaric oxygen treatment, but that exploration will be left to the reader. Some of these treatments have been well-researched and documented. Others haven't. Some have been FDA approved, others haven't.

Probably the individual survivor gets some of the best advice from other survivors who have received a treatment and benefited from it. However, keep in mind that each survivor's brain and stroke impact is different. What may work for one survivor may not work for another- including RAISE. However, we wish all stroke survivors the best of luck in whichever treatment they choose.

About the Author: Bob Guns

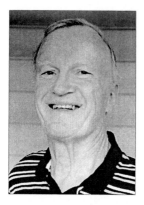

The author has practiced as teacher, school administrator, coach, lecturer, management trainer, business consultant, publisher, presenter, and author. Along the way, he acquired a Ph.D. and later on, a stroke that required brain surgery.

When initially recovering from his stroke, Bob asked why his life had been spared (about 80% of those who experienced a similar stroke died immediately). His answer? To prevent stroke and help stroke survivors: his new life purpose.

Beyond working on his own recovery, Bob started up a stroke support group in his community and acts as a 'You're the Cure' volunteer advocate at both the state and federal levels for the American Heart & Stroke Association.

Continuous learning guides Bob's life. His writing career spans business writing (a book, a chapter, and several articles); screenwriting; memoirs (over 70 unpublished pieces so far); and stroke articles published in 'Stroke Connection' magazine.

Bob currently resides (he has moved 35 times) in Mooresville, NC with his loving, supportive wife, Veronica and two mutually jealous shelties, Danny and Dixie. His son, Kevin, lives in Victoria, Canada, and his daughter, Laura (a model), resides on the most recent flight in or out of Charlotte.